See2See

Inland Sea
Road Trip

Publishing details

See2See 'Inland Sea' Road Trip
© 2020 Teresa Cutts, Gary R. Gunderson

ISBN 978-1-7324222-2-3

All profits from any sale of this book go to support the educational work of Stakeholder Health.

For information contact Stakeholder Health at:
www.StakeHolderhealth.org
or on Twitter at @stakehealth

Photographs in this book used with permission or from Gary Gunderson, Teresa Cutts, who hold their copyright.

Photo editing by Jim Cochrane using On1 RAW 2020.

Cover design & DTP: J. R. Cochrane
Map route extracted from Roadtrippers.com

See2See

Inland Sea

Road
Trip

Teresa Cutts
Gary R. Gunderson

ACKNOWLEDGEMENTS

As on the first trip, we owe the most thanks to those persons you'll meet later in the book—those at sites who generously gave of their precious time and insights about their work, and those liaisons who arranged these rich and diverse site visits along the way. We are particularly indebted to Jana Stoner of FaithHealth Appalachia in Huntington, West Virginia, Tim Allan of Cuyahoga County Board of Public Health, Heidi Gartland of University Health Systems in Cleveland, Peter Bath and PJ Brafford of Kettering Health Network in Dayton, and Jay Foster of Indiana University Health. These colleagues coordinated the bulk of our visits and journey, and we owe them special appreciation.

Stakeholder Health, the learning network of over 50 healthcare systems who care about partnerships with the vulnerable and marginalized in their communities, sponsored this trip; to the investing partners we offer a unique nod of gratitude.

Jeremy Moseley and Glenn Davis from Wake Forest Baptist Health joined us for certain legs of the journey and enriched the conversations. Jeremy also penned one of the blogs for the trip. Tom Peterson formatted and posted blogs along the way. Dawn Hall provided logistical support, without which none of the trip could have occurred. Robin Danner was a key copy editor for the piece, and Jim Cochrane provided the exquisite layout of the book.

Lastly, we wish to thank all our colleagues in the Wake Forest FaithHealth Division, who keep the work going on the ground while we wandered and learned through these trips— without their support and steady, high-quality work, this book would not be possible.

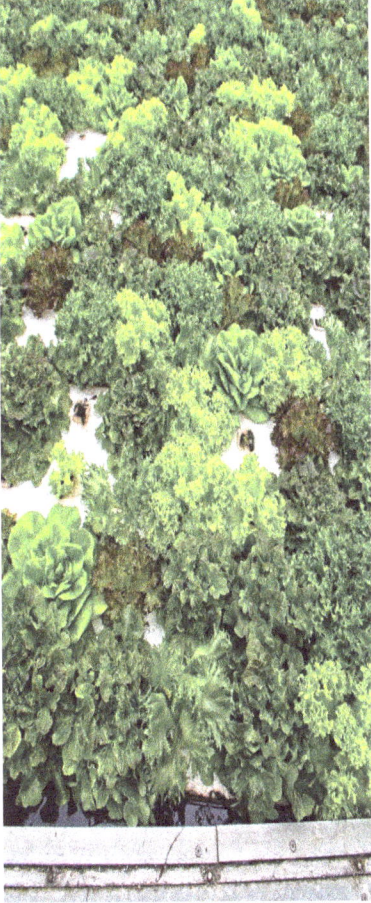

CONTENTS

Acknowledgements

Introduction   3

Monday, Nov. 18
      Huntington, W. Virginia   7

Tuesday, Nov. 19
      Cleveland, Ohio   35

Wednesday, Nov. 20
      Cleveland, Ohio   41

Thursday, Nov. 21
      Dayton, Ohio   54
      Indianapolis, Indiana   65

Friday, Nov. 22
      Indianapolis, Indiana   69
      Bloomington, Indiana   79

Endings and Beginnings   89

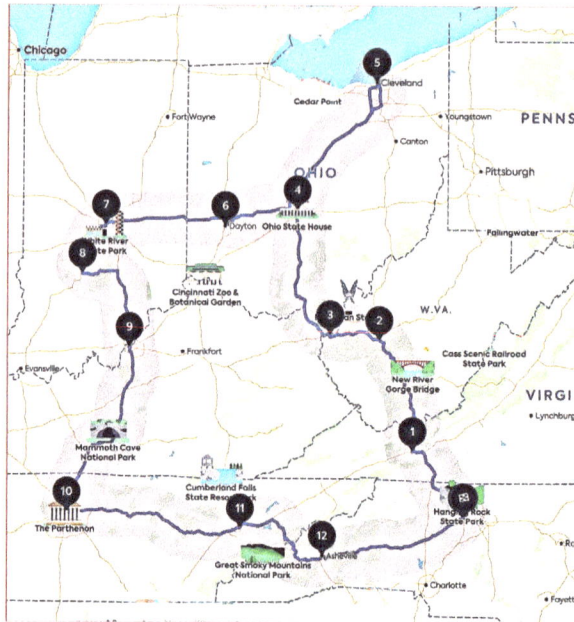

See2See 'Inland Sea' Visit Details

Huntington, W. Virginia

1- Leadership Breakfast, Cabell Huntington Hospital

2- Ebenezer Medical Outreach (EMO)

3- FaithHealth Appalachia Advisory Board, New Baptist Church

4- Provider Response Organization for Addiction Care & Treatment (PROACT)

5- Project Hope for Women and Children, Huntington City Mission

6- Quick Response Team (QRT), Real Life Christian Center Church

Cleveland, Ohio

7- Public Health, Health System & Community Partners Coalition, developing a CHNA, The Center for Health Affairs

8- Rainbow Babies & Children's Hospital

9- Evergreen Cooperatives

10- Cleveland Clinic, Pastoral Care and ACPE

Dayton, Ohio

11- Kettering Health System. Safety Net and Faith Community Partnerships, Grandview Hospital, Kettering

Indianapolis, Indiana

12- Near North West Faith Partners, Flanner House Community Center

13- Grassroots Maternal and Child Health Leadership Training Project: Riley Children's Foundation Infant Mortality Prevention Program

14- Shepherd Community Center

Bloomington, Indiana

15- Community Clinic at Redeemer Church, Monroe County FaithHealth Efforts

INTRODUCTION

Travelling the 'Inland Sea', learning on the road

Our second See2See Road Trip was designed to be less ambitious than going coast to coast, as we did in November 2018. This time we went up and around what the First People called the land below the Inland Sea. The trip promised to be quieter (no Winnebago), and eco-friendlier (we traded the Winnebago for a Mini-Cooper).

We expected less diversity than we saw on our inaugural 2018 cross-continental ride. Setting off across the West Virginia mountains on November 17th, 2019, heading for Huntington, West Virginia, seemed almost tame, although we knew that Huntington was the last thing from predictable. We were thankful to be back on the road in listening mode for a feast of learning, but glad for a more digestible, one week serving our purpose this time instead of earlier three.

However, this trip still surprised us in the depth of what we saw, heard and learned. Four themes began to emerge before lunch on the first stop in Huntington. *Places that have experienced perfect storms of trouble have also seen locals "holding on to one another through the storm"*. Second, *there is a transformation of compassion for the former "Others" that came out of those storms*. Third, we saw *a conviction by so many that "more has to be done to help" no matter what the issue and bravery in tackling the toughest of problems*. Lastly, and most importantly, we heard over and over again a return to *the notion that humans were the agents of the most pain upon others when it comes to Adverse Childhood Experiences and trauma BUT, that same human touch and relationship-building is the healing source for us all*.

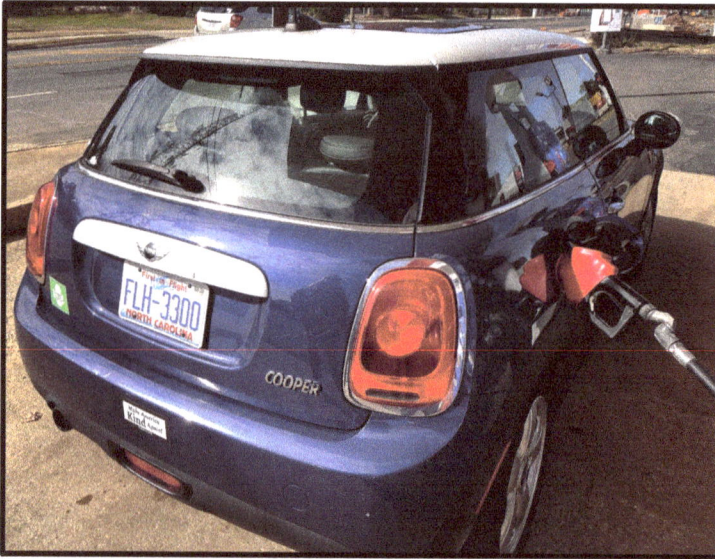

Gassing up the Trusty and Eco-Friendly Mini-Cooper in Winston-Salem

Relationship is the vehicle of both pain and healing. This is true regardless of whether a loved one has died, people are stuck in a job that doesn't fit or is toxic, live in ongoing poverty, have been jailed for drug use, had multiple overdoses, or are simply lonely. *Human connection, touch, and love are healing.* The simplest expression of compassion has power beyond any explanation. At the Quick Response Team meeting in Huntington, West Virginia, we heard the story of a person who opened the door to the Team a few days after his overdose: "You care enough to check up on *me*?" The peanut butter and jelly sandwich offered—along with condoms and treatment information—showed that the desire to help was real.

We began in Huntington, West Virginia, the former epicenter of the opioid crisis, now morphed into the "City of Solutions." What an apt, amazing new moniker! Their work with the Quick Response Team (including 31 mostly volunteer chaplains), the PROACT clinic for walk-ins seeking substance use disorder treatment, the Project Hope for Women and Children, and so much more, has helped decrease the overdose death rate by 50% in the past year. We were fed, as from a water hose, with a stream of information, passion, compassion and adaptability from the over 100 people we visited that first day.

Cleveland, on the shores of the Inland Sea itself, has many square miles of once-beautiful, now abandoned buildings. Tough people live here. We met with leaders from a brave and long-working collaborative group of public health, health system, and other partners who have managed to get almost all of the 22 hospitals in the county to do a joint Community Health Needs Assessment (CHNA), setting the near impossible standard of building trust and decreasing racism in their city. Terry Allen, the public health director, asked us to make him look boring, but he is quietly leading the County to declare structural racism a public health emergency.

Hospital leaders at University Health were most proud of their Rainbow Clinic for child and maternal care, for which they raised $40M in 16 months (their Board had thought there was no option of raising revenue). That clinic was designed by the local community and provides wrap around services on a nexus of two bus lines that has already resulted in neighborhood revitalization.

Next, we visited Evergreen Cooperatives, an employee owned cooperative in the heart of a formerly blighted neighborhood. The staff consist of a dedicated group of individuals, 55% of whom were formerly incarcerated. This is the icon of the Democracy Collaborative's "anchor institution" movement among hospitals. But the hospitals are the market, not the driver, for the best artisan hydroponic lettuce in the state. Evergreen now supplies 4,000 tons of locally grown basil every week for Nestle's research and development program. Chaplain Amy Greene from Cleveland Clinic updated us on their work, both inside and outside their internationally acclaimed walls.

Expecting a quiet morning with two or three spiritual care leaders from Kettering Health Network's hospital in Dayton, we found ourselves instead receiving another refreshing blast from the knowledge water hose, this time from our Stakeholder Health colleagues Peter Bath, PJ Brafford and 25 of their key local leaders.

Their extended family of community partners was grounded in faith, and ranged from Brigid's Path (for Neonatal Abstinence Syndrome babies and their Moms) to Frank Perez, Kettering's former system CEO's story. Frank shared how he received help in the cold winter of 1950's in Maryland from the Adventist run Good Neighbor House when he first immigrated to the States. Brigid's Path's CEO told emotionally of how God made a path for their ministry to thrive, including state legislation to support such care. Frank now serves as the Board Chair of the Dayton Good Neighbor House, who continues to evaluate and adapt the care they offer (lots of low-end and high-end dental and chronic care management) to meet the needs of their clients where they are. Primary Health Solutions, a local federally qualified health clinic, is now partnering intentionally with Kettering to fill the hole left by the closing of another hospital in the poorer section of town.

Indianapolis and Bloomington sparkle with excitement, their long-standing partnerships revitalized by Jay Foster (our former colleague from Wake Forest) coming into leadership there and receiving a large grant to create something akin to the Memphis Model and the North Carolina Way. Of particular interest were Shawn, the paramedic, and Adam, the police officer, working in a former high crime area near the Shepherd Center Community Center. Their work is all relational, whether getting air conditioning installed for a woman with respiratory problems, visiting a lonely woman who always seemed to call the ambulance on holidays, or interjecting tough love with a man with a severe alcohol problem.

It is common to think that highly challenged communities need lots of technical guidance in order for the locals to apply national-class best practices. We have long guessed that there is actually a great deal of technical competence widely dispersed in any community large enough to even think about a Starbucks. The communities finding their way against the tide have more than enough competence with which to work.

We should name a fifth theme that flowed through many, if not all, of our dozens of conversations: Spirit, or more, accurately, the *fruits* of the Spirit. There was rich diversity of faith persuasions and roles, but surprisingly little explicit theology. The fruits were clear, the deep roots felt: love, joy, peace, patience, kindness, humility, faithfulness, gentleness and self-control (Galatians 5:22). We were in a hurry to complete our 1,700-mile circuit and would need more time to fully grasp how these qualities emerged and then came to be offered with such generosity to their complex communities.

Monday, Nov. 18, 2019

Huntington, West Virginia

1. Leadership Breakfast, Cabell Huntington Hospital

https://www.cabellhuntington.org

Contacts: Jana Stoner, DMin, of FaithHealth Appalachia;
Deb Koester, PhD, Executive Director, West VA Local Health, Inc.

12 Attendees, 8 male, 4 female; All White

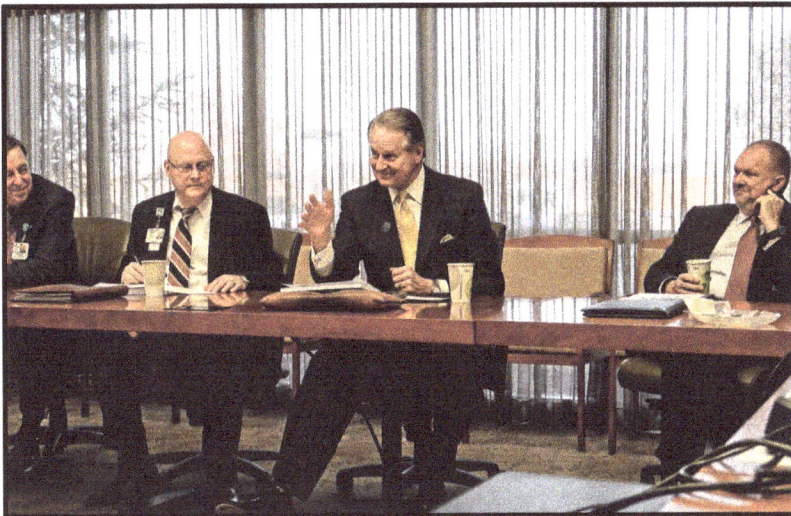

David Campbell, Hoyt Burdick, Steve Williams, Greg Creasy

We met with key leaders of Cabell Huntington Hospital (CHH) and the city, including Mayor Steve Williams, Mr. Kevin Fowler (CEO Cabell Huntington Hospital), Dr. Hoyt Burdick (CMO Mountain Health Network), Mr. David Campbell (Executive Director of Health Care Innovations), Dr. Jana Stoner (FaithHealth Appalachia), Ms. Jill Crawford (Executive Assistant), Ms. Kimberly Mallory (Director of Case Management at Cabell Huntington Hospital), Mr. Glen Thompson (Director of Care Management at St. Mary's Medical Center), Rev. Greg Creasy, (Director of Spiritual Care and Mission, St. Mary's), Rev. Tom Hastie, (Manager of Pastoral Care at CHH), Becky Bookwalter (Marketing Manager, Mountain Health Network), and a few others.

CEO Kevin Fowler introduced Mayor Steve Williams, whom he described as a "blessing to the community, innovative, passionate and a risk-taker." Mayor Williams offered a welcome and shared a rich and deep history of how Huntington went from being the epicenter of the opioid crisis to its current state, a "City of Solutions." He quoted Lao Tzu: "A leader is best when people barely know he exists; when his work is done, his aim fulfilled, they will say: 'we did it ourselves.'" He passionately shared his love of Huntington and he still wears a bracelet with the label "75." This refers to 75 persons who died in a crash when returning from a football game, now 49 years ago. He says that Huntington is a community that dealt with that crisis, economic downturns, crime and the subsequent opioid one by "Holding on to each other through the storms."

Huntington's citizens are connected, professionally and spiritually. The final straw came when shootings and crime came to what was once considered the better part of the city. A town hall meeting was held in which many stakeholders (law enforcement, public health, education, governmental, faith communities) said there was no "silver bullet" to combat the opioid epidemic. This enraged the Mayor and he encouraged all of the faith communities and more to pray together, starting with 5 key pastors. They created a raw video and e-mail and sent it out via these pastors (from the Pentecostal, Presbyterian, Baptist, Episcopalian, Non-Denominational groups, and more) and in less than a month had a million viewers.

On Sept. 7, 2014, he asked in the video for prayer to deliver Huntington from the epidemic, to protect first responders and deliver those caught up in addiction. He asked that people pray at 11:05 a.m. and this prayer request and prayer went out across the world. The Mayor added, laughingly, that, right after this, the rate of overdoses and addictions went up, but this started the momentum with leadership to create a different path, including those at Cabell Huntington Hospital (CHH).

Later, the mayor was then in Cleveland for a meeting, being interviewed by a reporter, who referred to Huntington as being the epicenter of the heroin epidemic in the U.S. But Mayor Williams thought that Huntington could become the "City of Solutions" with regard to the opioid epidemic. He believed that everyone in Huntington had an assignment, and he thought the city should name and own the problem. Cabell and St. Mary's (now Mountain Health) all stepped up, along with Marshall University, that now has a new Division of Addiction Science led by Dr. Stephen Petrany.

Now, from around the world people come to see what they have done and learned here. They are addressing prevention, intervention, family issues, economic concerns, forgiveness, and more. Lessons learned from years of work to move to the City of Solutions include the need to develop trust and create outcomes of hope, moving from brokenness to hope. He believes that hope isn't a strategy, it's an outcome.

Mayor Williams travels extensively and encourages other sites to look at their own assets and learn from Huntington, but to do the

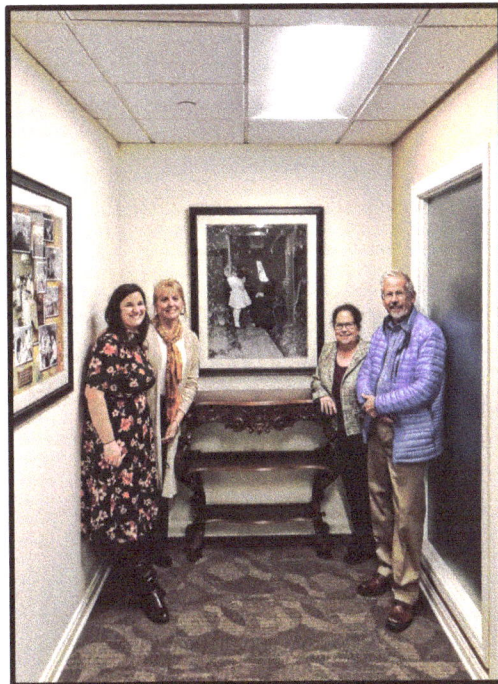

Jana Stoner, Pallottine Foundation's Janell Elizabeth Ray & Janet Spry, Gary Gunderson

work based on their own cultures and context. In Huntington, they repurposed persons, resources, assets, etc. For example, they worked with their Chief of the Fire Dept., a former nurse, data analyst, and the police chief in 2015 to develop a plan of action. They worked with the health systems to educate the community about and implement harm reduction approaches and learn about recovery models. Their approach is Interfaith, ranging from Christian to Muslim and even those who don't embrace traditional religious practice, because this is deeply spiritual work.

The timeline started in 2014, under Michael Botticelli (Office of Drug Control and Policy) in the Obama administration. However, in 2016, Fentanyl hit the streets and the rate of overdoses soared. A critical turning point was August 15, 2016, when 26 people overdosed in 4 hours; 2 of them died. They realized that saving someone from dying from an overdose in that moment was not saving them in the long run, especially if they weren't referred to treatment. On Sept. 12, 2016, Ms. Taylor Wilson (who had been among those 26) died, two days before she was accepted into a suboxone treatment program.

First Responders went to Colerain, OH, and learned about their Quick Response Team (QRT) program, in which a paramedic, law enforcement officer, and recovery coach went within 72 hours to visit a person who overdosed, to encourage treatment and help in any way. Huntington added pastors to the team and now 31 volunteer pastors rotate call on the QRT. Their overdose rates dropped 40% from 2017 to 2018. They received a $1.6M HHS Dept. of Justice grant to help with Compassion fatigue and a $1M Bloomberg grant for technical assistance. Becky Bookwalter, of Connect through Caring Compassion from Mountain Health, had just finished the 2016 CHNA and didn't want to just check off the box.

There were six health priorities, and two over-arching goals: behavioral health and substance use disorder, particularly neonatal abstinence syndrome (NAS); and the prevention and management of chronic diseases, like diabetes, heart disease, obesity and more.

So, with Kevin Fowler's help, they arranged to hold a Health Summit in June 2016, focused on all 23 counties across the three states (West Virginia, Ohio, Kentucky) that constituted Cabell Huntington's catchment area. Representatives from hospitals across the region showed up for the Summit and the response was anything but perfunctory. There was a desire to create changes in health at a different scope and scale. They've now held three Summits, with ever increasingly expert key speakers, even the current Surgeon General of the USA.

From the first Summit came PROACT, a collaborative clinic focused on management and treatment of substance use disorder (SUD), FaithHealth Appalachia, mentoring in the ED for persons with SUD, and so much more. These programs were built and paid for from recovery funds. Huntington found talent "hiding in plain sight," like Jan Radar, the current Chief of the Fire Department, the first female Fire Chief in the state and also a nurse. She was named to *Time's* 100 most influential persons in the world list this year and has given an inspiring Ted Talk (this is available at https://www.insider.com/west-virginia-fire-chief-jan-rader-opioid-epidemic-ted-talk). Under her watch from the 2017 baseline, overdoses decreased 40% and overdose deaths by 50%.

Dr. Hoyt Burdick, Chief Clinical Officer at Mountain Health Network, shared the history of the two hospitals that have chosen to join together to create a higher level of care for the 26-county service area. The recent merger resulted in the creation of the Pallottine Foundation in Huntington in 2017. Dr. Burdick told us that the Pallottine Sisters' order of nuns came to Huntington in 1924. Interestingly, all had had bookings on the Titanic, but one sister's papers were not in order, so they opted not to take the ship (with good consequences!). They were the chief leaders that helped start St. Mary's Health System. Starting in 1945, the State planned to open the Cabell Huntington Charitable Hospital, but due to lags in the legislature, it finally opened only in 1955. The Sisters created a call for community-based care that was centered on Christ. Mountain Health (now the umbrella health system joining CHH and St. Mary's) had a mission of connecting a higher level of care, so their two missions aligned well.

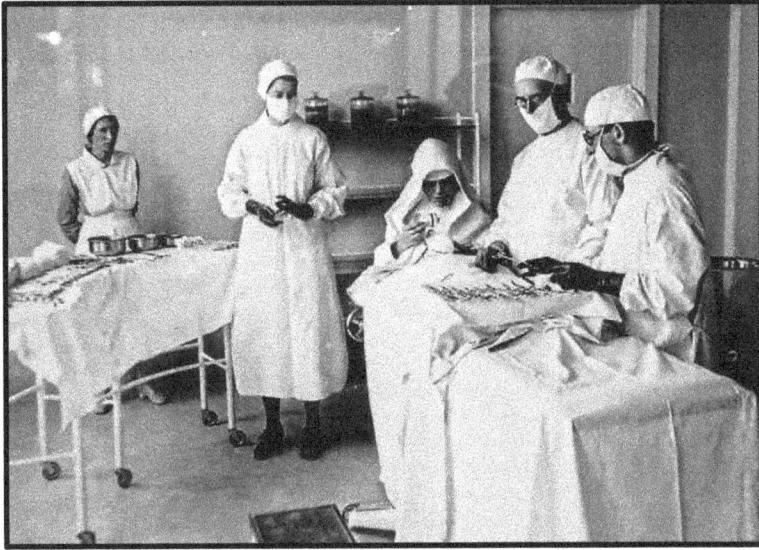

St. Mary's Hospital Sisters and Staff

In the 1970's, veterans were not being well served, so a new medical school, Marshall University, was established. A new Veterans Administration hospital was also established in Huntington, which was conveniently located on the old CNO railroad line. Marshall University moved into the old CNO hospital, which before had served the Ivy League, robber baron types and physicians. Since that time, this blue-collar school of medicine has become world-renowned for its new Addiction Science Medicine Department and its community-based, innovative approaches to combating the opioid crisis in West Virginia. They study compassion fatigue in first responders, decreasing stigma around SUD, and much more.

Drawing from experts and their models, Huntington has made a difference in decreasing opioid use and deaths. Dr. Terry Horton, from Christiana Health System in Delaware, has an inpatient focus beyond just withdrawal, adding active treatment efforts while persons are hospitalized long-term for treatment of endocarditis or other medical problems secondary to drug use. Dr. Gail D'Onofrio's (Yale) emergency room assessment has also been used, successfully. Their Opioid Work Group studies the results of these practices and has identified numerous quality metrics, monitored via the collaborative CHNA partnership.

Dave Campbell, Executive Director of Health Care Innovations, stated that as they embrace Population Health work, they are relying on the models developed by Stakeholder Health, the American Hospital Association, and IHI's Pathways to Population Health or P2PH (particularly the fourth domain of bio-psycho-social-spiritual health). The question is not just "How we care for you?" but "Do we care about you?" The wholistic view of the individual is important, as is meeting people where they are. There is a focus on the family as well. Community health and well-being is improving in Huntington to the extent that it is now being termed the "Community of Solutions."

2. Ebenezer Medical Outreach (EMO)

http://www.emohealth.org/

Contacts: Rebecca Glass, Executive Director of EMO;
Dr. Matthew Christiansen, Medical Director
8 Attendees. 2 males, 6 females; 6 White, 2 AA

Ebenezer Medical Outreach or EMO provides access to affordable and free, comprehensive health care, preventative care, and pharmaceuticals to underserved persons in the Fairfield West community of Huntington and the surrounding areas. They are guided by a system of beliefs recognizing health care as a basic right to which all are entitled.

Rebecca Glass, Executive Director and Women's Health Coordinator of EMO, led us on a tour of the clinic. The clinic was repurposed from its old use as a high school in the area. Their Women's Clinic provides nutrition supplements and teaches participants how to feed a family of four on $4 per day and $28 per week. Medications are provided via the

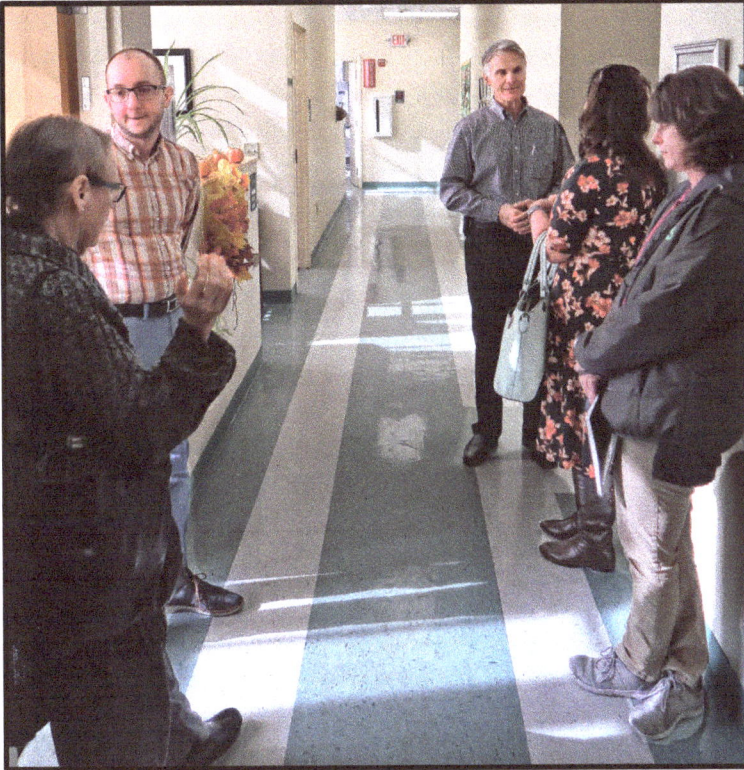

Donna Rumbaugh, Matthew Christiansen, Glenn Davis,
Jana Stoner, Christy Fawcette

patient assistance program. Their Dental Clinic is free as well and the EMO provides care for both the uninsured and under-insured with high deductibles.

All persons must be approved by the Dept. of Health and Human Resources (DHHR) to obtain EMO services and are issued an EMO card. To be vetted as eligible for services, persons must have a denial letter from Medicaid via the DHHR. They do receive some uncompensated care money from the state, as well as funding from Adult & Senior services. Marshall University provides billing services, as well as both Family Practice and pharmacy staff (lead pharmacist and pharmacy technician). They ask for a minimum donation of $3 for services and many medical staff are trained here.

Dr. Matthew Christiansen has been the Medical Director for the past year and trained here himself as a resident. Like many states, the number of free clinics in West Virginia is declining, with the plan that expanded Medicaid would decrease the need for them. However, there is still a need for free clinic services, as many of their clients work several part-time, low-paying jobs, and have no health insurance coverage. EMO provides wrap around care, has sub-specialty clinics in orthopedics, and also provides an annual eye clinic where persons can be screened and obtain eyeglasses for $30.

Diagnostically, the state Breast and Cervical Cancer Screening Program (BCCSP) helps, but they have a need for more colonoscopies. Both hospitals and Marshall University help a lot, donating staff, x-rays, and routine blood work. They struggle to show their true Return on Investment in terms of quantifying the amount of uncompensated care provided. Many of their providers are volunteers, including a dental hygienist, a community dentist, and medical providers who are retirees.

EMO started in 1996, as a branch of the church. Dr. Christiansen does this work because it is rewarding personally and helps remind him of his initial reason to work in medicine: to help others, especially the under-served. Also, working at EMO helps him step away from the more technical and instrumental parts of medical practice in other sites, like meeting patient quotas and billing numbers to show productivity. Here at EMO, he can take time to focus on improving the world, one patient at a time.

Likewise, residents see what the lives of under-served persons are like and the work gets them back to providing for the basics and learning what can be done within the limited resources and constrained environment of this clinic. The former department chair in Internal Medicine at Marshall University was the previous Medical Director at EMO, which accounts for its strong support.

EMO does screening for HIV/AIDS. It works closely with the local needle exchange and harm reduction coalitions at the Cabell Huntington Health Department. Although they haven't seen an upsurge in HIV/AIDS caused by IV drug use (last year the new infection numbers went from 80 to 81), nearby southern Indiana has seen those numbers shoot up to 1,500 people over the past two years.

Five years ago, EMO saw a spike in the new Hepatitis C infections, but now Medicaid is covering that costly anti-viral treatment, so rates are

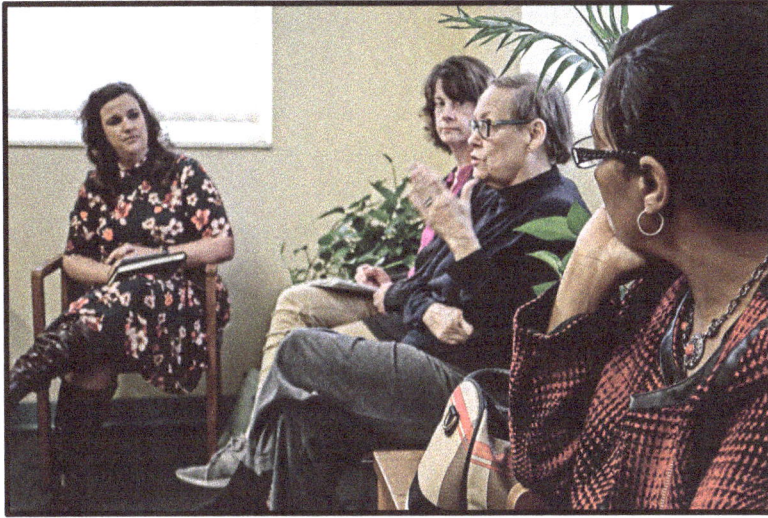
Jana Stoner and Connectors Christy Fawcette, Donna Rumbaugh and Teresa Johnson

good. Medicaid also provides good coverage for substance abuse screening, physician visits and medically assisted treatment.

Faith Communities were previously reluctant to help with substance use disorder (SUD) but now, with so many congregations impacted, everyone is willing to help. Donna Rumbaugh, the West End Connector for FaithHealth Appalachia, shared about this and her frustration in some church members' past judgmental natures. In the past, traditional church practice was feeding Thanksgiving Dinner to the poor or marginalized, but members were often afraid of those in recovery.

Now that has changed. The number of grandparents in church raising their own grandchildren due to the parents' addiction is rising dramatically. One local parsonage in the West End neighborhood is a recovery house. Three-quarters of the 60 members are in some form of recovery. The Regional Health Connects program has been useful and Donna now understands that she must be respectful of all persons' views and feelings about SUD, as they have their reasons.

A big focus from the council now is raising awareness and providing education about SUD, as well as decreasing underage vaping. Currently, there are an estimated 10K children in West Virginia engaged in vaping. The opportunity for faith communities to help with community lament/grieving to deal with overdose losses was noted.

The Quick Response Team (QRT) visits homes after overdoses and/or overdose deaths and brings a clergy person as a regular part of their team, offering that pastoral care.

EMO also offers chronic care management, with many patients having multiple comorbidities. They train residents about the limitations that under-served patients have in making the best choices for dealing with diabetes and other problems. Many lack the time to exercise, lack money to eat healthy foods, and may be working several jobs, so they feel too tired to engage in exercise to decrease stress and improve overall health status.

Matthew has become proficient at Motivational Interviewing, a short-term type of counseling to meet people where they are in the stages of behavior change (pre-contemplation, contemplation, preparation, activity, maintenance, and relapse). This may trigger a conversation that is more useful and tailored to the individual. He rarely has time to insert basic nutritional knowledge or physical education (e.g., how processed food is not healthy or real food, ways to exercise more in daily life). A team approach is needed for that and the local Agricultural Extension has classes on canning vegetables, fruit, and even meat, which can be a huge benefit, especially for persons in more rural areas.

Dr. Christensen's wife is the local City Planner and Huntington itself is moving toward more community wellness. A local senator, Paul Ambrose, died in one of the 9-11 crashes and there is a new walking trail named after him that allows biking and walking more easily. Community gardens are springing up.

Resiliency and wellness training for first responders is a focus, to give them outlets for their emotional responses. Teresa Johnson, the Fairfield Connector for FaithHealth Appalachia, also shared a story illustrating EMO's great work. EMO's clinical and other services were lauded by a former patient (and now Recovery Coach) with Type I diabetes, who said that EMO's offerings saved him. Christy Fawcette, the High Lawn Connector for FaithHealth Appalachia, also was positive about EMO's services.

3. FaithHealth Appalachia Advisory Board, New Baptist Church

http://www.newbaptistchurch.com/

Contacts: Jana Stoner, DMin of FaithHealth Appalachia; Dr. Trent Eastman, New Baptist Church

24 Attendees, 18 male, 6 female; 22 White, 2 AA

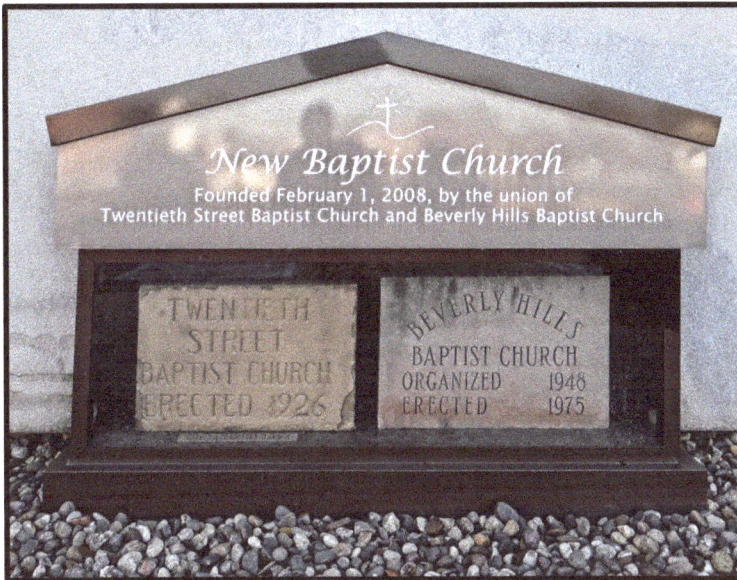

Twin Stones at the New Baptist Church

On-route to this meeting, Jana Stoner, Director of FaithHealth Appalachia, offered a driving tour and brief history of the Highlawn neighborhood in Huntington. It got its name from its literal "high lawn" on the banks of the Ohio River, so high that no flood wall was needed there to protect properties. Once a thriving business, industry and residential blue-collar area, it hosted most of the city's industry, including where railroad cars were built, as well as many schools. After many industries left the area, the neighborhood was distressed and twenty years ago, several schools, including the large Huntington East High School and Enslow Middle School, closed.

One church, Highlawn Baptist Church, had a membership of up to 1,500 persons and was the hub for social services in the community, providing food baskets and other goods to those in need. Infighting in the church resulted in a church split between the Southern and American Baptist factions. Nine years ago, the church was down to 25 members, so it closed and sold its building to St. Mary's Medical Center, leaving a huge void in the community.

In recent years, this building has provided community worship space for several Highlawn churches to gather to worship alongside one another. Initially, starting in 1924, the Pallotine Sisters worked in the Highlawn area, due to great need. At that time, St. Mary's Medical Center was started but not seen as a huge asset by local residents. Many locals perceived it as shutting down their roads and buying up their properties. A new Pallotine Foundation of Huntington has been in operation for about two years now, resulting from the merger between St. Mary's Health System and Cabell Huntington Hospital.

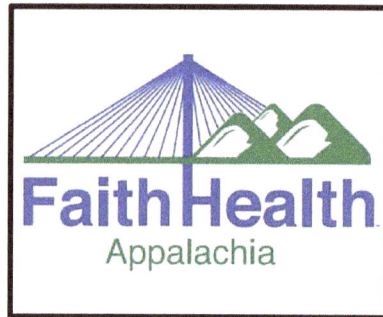

Jana Stoner's father was a Surgical Physician Assistant and they moved to Huntington when she was ten years old. She has a deep love for the city and the Highlawn neighborhood. She believes that both faith communities and health systems need to be more accountable in terms of care in their city. The beginnings of collaborative work were there when she and her husband came back to the city in 2006. Both had been serving as ministers, she as a children's minister and he as youth minister. Now her husband is the Chief Operating Officer at a company serving as the hub of social enterprise in Southern West Virginia. They provide housing, agriculture, woodworking and other training as part of a coal miner workforce development program—33 hours of work, 6 hours community care, and 3 hours personal development.

Through Jana's Doctor of Ministry work, the local churches still in this neighborhood have now banded together to provide care in that space, and on November 24, 2019, they had their second annual collaborative worship in the former High Lawn Baptist church. This alliance also raised $50K together to help build a Habitat for Humanity house and leveraged $200K to help rebuild the community. As such, Jana was a perfect choice to take on the leadership of FaithHealth Appalachia when that role emerged. Developing a stronger FaithHealth collaboration in Huntington, including Fairfield, Healthy Highlawn and West End neighborhoods, is one of their goals.

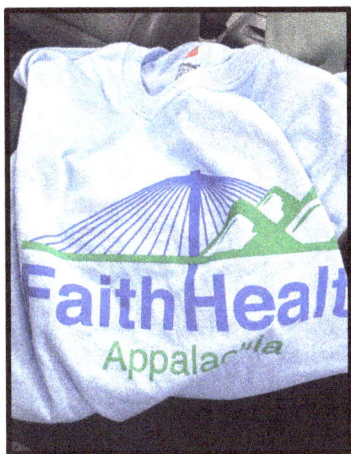
FaithHealth Appalachia T-shirt

At New Baptist, Pastor Trent Eastman gave a quick tour and history of the congregation. New Baptist was a blending of a new church (Beverly Hills Baptist) and an older one (20th Street Baptist) that was closing in 2008. They took over an empty ice-skating rink and used it for the new blended congregation's space in Highlawn. Trent also teaches at Palmer Seminary but serves as Senior Pastor at New Baptist.

The FaithHealth Appalachia Board was well-represented by denominational leaders of all types: Baptists, Assembly of God, Church of the Nazarene, United Methodist Church, Lutheran, Catholic, Episcopalian. FH Appalachia set three goals for 2019. First, they established infrastructure, via developing by-laws, hiring a Director and three Connectors, and identifying a referral process at both hospitals (CHH and St. Mary's) to address six areas of the social determinants of health, as well as identify if a person had a primary care provider. They are keeping track of data via electronic medical records when persons touch the hospitals, doing 7, 14, 21 and 28-day check-ins after initial visits.

They are also building infrastructure to promote wholistic health community wide. They hosted a Pastor Appreciation Lunch that was attended by 80 pastors, with 100 churches from Huntington alone represented. Wellness events are being held and ties are being strengthened with Faith Community Nurses across all three states of West Virginia, Ohio and Kentucky. These events focus on substance use disorder, Adverse Childhood Experiences, disaster preparedness and diabetes prevention. Marshall University staff has provided help with a community health worker model that focuses on intense chronic care management.

Chaplain Tom Hastie shared that FH Appalachia, from the CHH perspective, was driven by the "Lord, not hospital-owned," and that Jana's doctoral work laid tracks for the initiative to succeed. Tom called Jana the "spark plug" that the work needed. Another dynamic in its success, as they see it, is that God put together clergy and other leaders who already had organic relationships established, which is the glue of the work. Pastor Fred McCarty, from Walnut Hills Church of the Nazarene, said that the Board's initial question of how the clergy and congregations could connect into hospitals was answered by "God's perfect storm" to address the needs of the opioid crisis and the already existing assets and relationships locally.

The Quick Response Team or QRT (now with 31 trained and mostly volunteer clergy) is a good example of fruit of God's perfect storm. The diverse clergy transcend theological differences by keeping the work God Christ-Centered, and focusing on "God's Plan", not people's plan. Jana's leadership to encourage churches to collaborate has been helpful, by asking all congregations to pray for one another's success. Now, there is a weekly prayer meeting for clergy to pray and love collaboratively. This has been energizing for many churches. Pastor Deb Winters of the Transformation Community Church is now "on fire" with love and caring for the community.

Pastor Trent Eastman shared that there are two agendas. One is that of the hospital or corporate agenda, to decrease readmissions and unnecessary emergency room visits; this doesn't resonate with the churches. The second agenda is more of what FH Appalachia embraces: how one can support and build up the churches, by equipping each church to be part of God's work in the community (not just meet hospital needs/wants). Chaplain Glenn Creasy says that they have had to adapt Memphis and FH North Carolina's models to their particular organic assets and relationships. Interestingly, at the start of FH Appalachia, they had all attendees to draw a picture of what they thought the initiative would look like. The pictures were all totally different, but they have settled on bridge building as an iconic and appropriate symbol. Bringing public health into FH Appalachia's work is great for all.

4. Provider Response Organization for Addiction Care & Treatment (PROACT)

www.proactwv.org

Contact: Dr. Beth Welsh
11 Attendees, 4 males, 7 females; 10 White, 1 AA

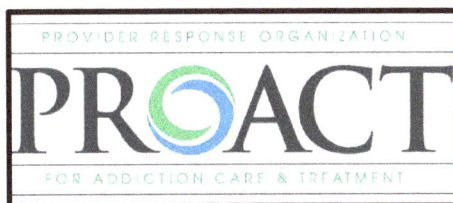

Provider Response Organization for Addiction Care & Treatment, or PROACT, is an outpatient medical facility that serves as a single regional referral point to assess patients following discharge from local emergency rooms and inpatient detox units, and by referral from its quick response teams and other emergency medical response teams. PROACT also accepts self-referrals and referrals from community providers.

The ultimate goal is to effectively serve, educate and treat individuals through and beyond the initial stages of recovery until they become long-term, committed members of society. PROACT is a collaborative effort of Marshall Health, Cabell Huntington Hospital, St. Mary's Medical Center, Thomas Health System and Valley Health.

PROACT provides individuals with substance use disorders and their families with a viable system that provides positive outcomes. The center functions as a centralized hub for treatment, recovery, therapy, education, research, workforce opportunities, and support for those affected by addiction. PROACT improves and increases access for patients and providers dealing with substance use disorder as well provides the necessary support for community physicians treating patients with the disorder.

PROACT's building was an old renovated CVS drugstore. Opening on Oct. 21, 2018, the program is a collaboration between Mountain Health (Cabell Huntington Hospital or CHH and St. Mary's Medical Center), Thomas Health System, and Valley Health. The two local hospitals' initial monetary gift of $1.4M paid for the renovation of the building. CHH holds the lease on the building. Thomas Health System, out of Charleston, and Valley Health, provide medication-assisted treatment (MAT) with suboxone and vivitrol.

PROACT is a merged, federally qualified, behavioral health center and MAT clinic, with multiple collaborators and partnerships. It was born out of Huntington's leaders' frustration and broken hearts caused by so many opioid deaths. Referrals come from individuals, courts and families, and PROACT aims to be easy to find and access, often with same day initial assessments.

Their first patient was a woman living in a nearby crack house, who had lost custody of her children. Unfortunately, after she enrolled, she then dropped out of the program. PROACT currently sees about 500 people per week, averaging 86 intakes per month, now with over 1,000 intakes of record. 86% of their clients are on heroin, while most of the others use methamphetamines. After assessment, providers help persons craft plans for detoxification, and intensive outpatient or residential addiction treatment. About 67% of their patients are covered by Medicaid. They also get some philanthropy, but all profits are rolled back into sustaining the program.

PROACT offers individual group therapy, patient navigators, and peer support and spiritual care. Chaplain Rodney Adkins, who started in August, helps clients identify and put into practice ways to get and stay clean. He believes that connection to others and self and whoever you see as a 'Higher power' is crucial to achieve abstinence. Addiction detaches people from others and from goals and leaves a void. He believes that absence of connection leads to addiction and intently tries to listen twice as much as he talks. He also runs weekly family support meetings, advocates for positive reinforcement, and focuses on educating local faith leaders about substance use disorders. He leads tours of PROACT for local community leaders to demystify what occurs there.

Michael Haney, Executive Director of PROACT, outlines three factors that make the program unique: multi-agency and stakeholder collaboration, spiritual care, and how they deal with physicians who do this work. The clinic has eight prescribers who alternate half day shifts to avoid burnout and are paid flat fees. They are truly only limited by space in terms of how many persons they see. Walk-in care is often arranged, for primary care or basic mental health needs.

Their reputation for getting persons to care quickly has spread. One woman, who was living in St. Louis and relapsed, was given a bus ticket to Huntington by her church, which knew she could receive great care at PROACT. Their services could be viewed as concierge or tourism addiction medical treatment.

Many PROACT staff are cross-trained. Michael himself does assessments. In terms of their relationship with faith communities, there have been meetings with the Black Pastors Association, tours of the program, talks at churches, and a second year Clinical Pastoral Care resident was based there who is now their full-time chaplain. They work closely with the local harm reduction and needle syringe program, receiving referrals, and have their residents work with PROACT as well.

Michael has been amazed at the cooperation in the city to focus on a solution to the opioid crisis. They work with CHH's counseling center and have pediatric chaplains from Lilly's Place (for neonatal abstinence syndrome babies). PROACT also partners with West Virginia's regional jail treatment programs in terms of discharge planning as people leave incarceration. There are many community-based chaplaincy residency programs, including St. Mary's Employee Assistance Program (EAP) for first responders and a chaplain for first responders at COMPASS.

When PROACT first opened there were some mixed community responses. Many neighbors felt that they had no choice in where the clinic was placed. The stigma around those with addictions is still high. Many locals walk together in groups of two or three to get to the clinic (also called "trudging to treatment"), which bothers some neighbors. Michael and others are working on opening dialogue with them and both repairing and building trust.

5. Project Hope for Women and Children; Huntington City Mission

https://www.huntingtoncitymission.org/project-hope/

Contact: Jessica Tackett, Program Director, Project Hope for Women & Children; Terri Gogus, Therapist for Project Hope

2 Attendees, 2 White females

Project Hope for Women and Children welcomed its first family on December 26, 2018. An 18-unit residential treatment facility in downtown Huntington, West Virginia, Project Hope is designed to meet the specific needs of mothers working to overcome substance use disorder. As a comprehensive treatment facility, Project Hope bridges a gap in the continuum of care by providing onsite peer and residential support around the clock, life skills training and mental health services.

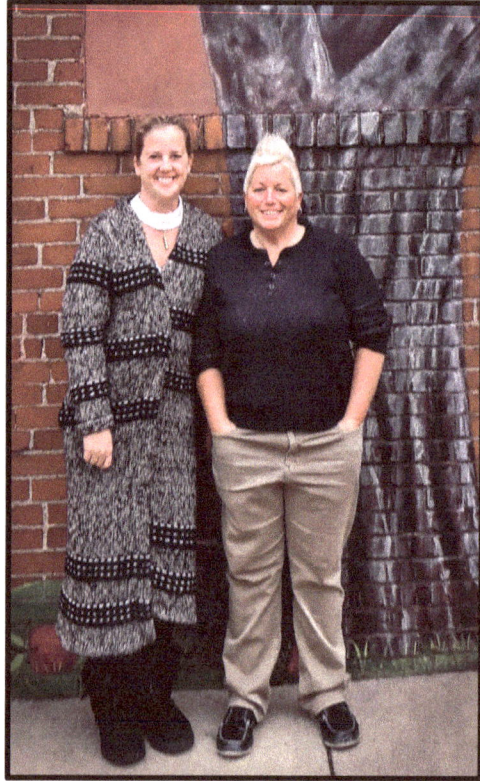
Project Hope's Jessica Tackett and Terry Gogus

The building now occupied by Project Hope once served as a transitional living complex for the homeless on the corner of 7th Avenue and 10th Street. After a $1.8 million renovation by Marshall Health in 2018, each apartment has either two or three bedrooms, one bathroom, a large living area, and lots of closets. The units are fully furnished, with television and internet. Mothers overcoming addiction can bring up to four children with them during the course of their treatment program, which averages about 6 months.

Caring for women with substance use disorder is something the Marshall University Joan C. Edwards School of Medicine and Marshall Health have been doing in their clinics and teaching hospitals for nearly a decade. This newest initiative, Project Hope for Women and Children, partners with the Huntington City Mission, as well as other community resources, such as the Provider Response Organization for Addiction Care & Treatment (PROACT), RV CARES (Center for Addiction Research and Support), Cabell Huntington Hospital, and Healthy Connections, to take that care to the next level.

The cornerstone of Project Hope is person-centered care. That means each client's treatment plan is specific to her situation. Treatment options include access to off-site abstinence-based and medication-assisted treatment (MAT) if needed, group and individual therapy, and transportation. The program's two 12-passenger vans transport clients to and from health care, social security, jobs, child care, legal and other appointments including AA or NA meetings. Many of the women have been court-ordered to treatment. A number have also given birth while in the program. Project Hope staff act as the client's advocate throughout the entire journey.

Perhaps one of the most unique things about Project Hope is that it focuses on the family unit. Family support includes family therapy, unification with children, and community support. To see if they are meeting developmental milestones, children's motor skills, speech, hearing, and vision are assessed in a Kids Clinic. Before clients graduate, they are connected to permanent housing, a job, and other resources to help them transition smoothly. Project Hope staff work with clients to help them sign up for SNAP benefits and connect them with programs like West Virginia WORKS and Creating Opportunities for Recovery Employment (CORE) to build job skills and secure permanent employment after treatment.

Among the program's 16 staff, Program Director Jessica Tackett leads the day-to-day operations at Project Hope. Jessica was in the military and has worked as an alcohol and drug counselor and suicide prevention officer. Terri Gogus is a therapist (licensed clinical social worker) who formerly worked for the Bureau for Behavioral Health. Additional staff, all of whom must, as Jessica puts it, have "love, patience, empathy and a passion to do the work," include two family navigators, a recovery coach, a driver and many key volunteers. The Huntington community has embraced both the concept and clients at Project Hope. Volunteers provide programming and meals on site, as well as informal mentoring and babysitting. They host pampering events for the moms and baby showers for new additions to the Project Hope family.

Recovery, however, is hard and sometimes the process requires "tough love." Relapses happen, even in a strict, high-intensity residential environment. Project Hope has had to discharge three clients because of verbal or physical altercations with staff. But, even then, the staff stays in touch with them.

The "wins" are always worth the battle. "When you see that spark happen for that mother, it is like no other feeling," Jessica said. The emotional intensity of the environment can leave staff both mentally and emotionally exhausted, so Project Hope stresses good self-care for staff, including caring for one another.

So far, 13 women have completed the treatment program at Project Hope. Many of the graduates have stayed connected, which also aids them in their recovery. Eight graduates have come back to teach Zumba classes or join in holiday celebrations. Project Hope remains their home away from home.

Funding for Project Hope comes through Medicaid reimbursements for clinical services, grants from the U.S. Substance Abuse and Mental Health Administration and the West Virginia Department of Health and Human Resources as well as private donors. They also receive a per diem rate from the State for adults served.

Telling the story of Project Hope's excellent work is a delicate matter due to the stigma still associated with substance use disorder and because staff want to protect the privacy of their clients and their children. Some narratives have been published in local newspapers, but they are careful always to protect the names and privacy of those they serve.

6. Quick Response Team (QRT), Real Life Christian Center Church

http://www.cityofhuntington.com/assets/pdf/document-center/QRT_Brochure.pdf

Contact: Mrs. Connie Priddy
24 Attendees, 18 male, 6 female; 18 White, 6 AA

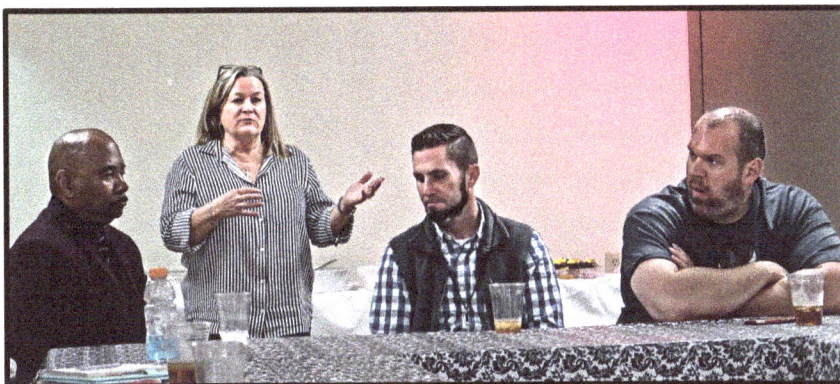

Virgil Johnson, Connie Priddy, Duane Little, Ben Howard

The Quick Response Team (QRT) visits individuals in the community 24 to 72 hours after they have experienced an overdose, to meet people where they are, show up, be vulnerable, and engage in a discussion of treatment opportunities. The Huntington QRT is the only one in the country that includes a faith leader as part of the team. A member of the EMS, a certified peer recovery coach, and law enforcement are additional members of the team. In Cabell County this year, overdoses are down more than 40%. More and more people are receiving treatment because many people are showing up with a consistent message … you matter. You are important. You are loved. You are a child of God. You are not alone.

We met with the Huntington QRT at the church of Bishop C.D. Shaw, the Real Life Christian Center, which is located in a more underserved part of the city. Their QRT includes Team Lead Larrecsa Cox, of the EMS, Ben Howard of the police department, whom some call "Big Ben," and Kenny Sargent, a peer support specialist in recovery, with a rotating staff of 31 trained pastors who all take turns making visits in the community. Bishop Shaw did initial visits and now creates the clergy schedule for the team. Connie Priddy, QRT program director, based at the Cabell County EMS, shared that she was born and raised in Huntington and watched in horror as Huntington had become the "epicenter of the opioid crisis" in 2016. The crisis came to a head when 26 persons overdosed within a few hours then, and none of those persons had been referred for treatment.

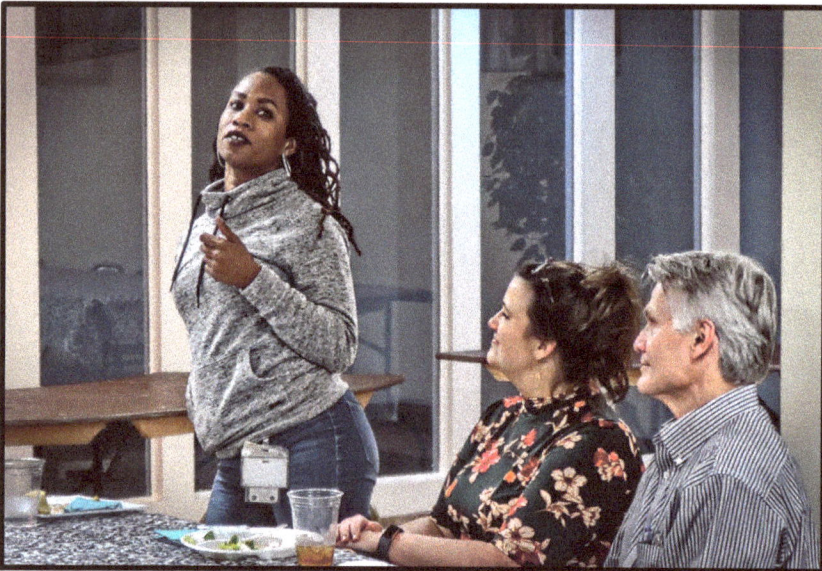

Larrecsa Cox, Jana Stoner, Glenn Davis

Huntington leaders looked for a solution and went to learn about a model used in nearby Colerain, OH, near Cincinnati. The Colerain QRT visited people and/or families left behind if the person died within a few days of the event, and they had achieved an 80% rate of persons going to treatment after the QRT visit. Huntington started their visits even though there was no additional funding and the city was struggling financially.

So the team made 30 informal visits for "love, not money" in the first half of 2017. Fortunately, a Federal large grant was awarded in Oct. 2017 and they began their work in earnest by the end of December 2017. Their baseline metric was the number of ambulance overdose calls, which at that time were well over 2,000, averaging at least 6 per day.

Huntington's QRT wondered how persons who overdosed would receive their visits. Would they be combative? Certainly, many were embarrassed. The generally positive response to their visits, however, was found in the poignant question of a man who they visited, post-overdose, who said, "You care enough to check up on me?" Those visited could feel the authenticity and caring of real people reaching out. Ninety-eight percent of the time their visits are received in a positive and non-confrontational way.

The QRT knew they wanted to include the faith community in this new opportunity to reach out into the community. The Huntington Area Black Pastors Ministerial Association was approached and asked how they could help with neighbors who were addicted. QRT asked for food, clothing, a safe place for meeting, etc. Bishop Shaw said, "No, we want to go with the team and do something more meaningful."

So now, two years later, clergy have been trained and are showing up and going with the team regularly, with no gaps in that service. All other team members truly value the clergy's presence and help, and they all comfort and care for one another. Often, the team members get to know those who may ultimately die of an overdose, which is hard for them all. As Larrecsa says, "Some persons really touch our hearts."

The QRT has no set script. When they find a person (at homes, parks, cars, on the street), the team looks to see with whom the person makes eye contact first. That team member moves into a lead role, often like a jazz ensemble. The team have great relationships and sees their work as very grassroots. They believe that first responders should be the point of first contact, but then link the person visited to harm reduction, a primary care provider, or set up testing for HIV/AIDS and/or treatment.

Larrecsa sees their work as more like social work, as many people need the basics: housing, food, a phone, transportation, etc. They have been able to bring many of those services to the persons visited, like a local HIV/AIDS interventional specialist who is now doing Rapid Testing in the field. The team also started making peanut butter sandwiches, filling brown bags with those, condoms, information on substance use disorder (SUD) treatment and other resource listings, as well as a purple rubber bracelet with the QRT's number on it, for ease of access.

Every workday offers something different and they all learn something new each day. The subtle aspects of caring for those with SUD are immense. Even if a person wants to go for treatment, do they have Medicaid coverage or transportation to Charleston? Do they need food in the short-run? The QRT enrolls people in Medicaid and obtains medication cards, and gets them to medical professionals if they have endocarditis due to drug use and/or other health problems. They go to jails to meet with those whom they have developed relationships in the community, and to the mothers and fathers and family members of those with SUD who call for help for their loved one.

The QRT helps with all these needs and processes. They have even been called on to "dog sit" for persons heading to treatment. Larrecsa admits, sheepishly, that six months later she still has one person's dog. The Charleston QRT has established a Pet Refuge for this purpose. Needless to say, setting boundaries can be problematic with the intensity of this work. However, the QRT's mantra is "helping people where they are." They are not there to judge or shame or blame, just help.

Kenny, the peer support recovery specialist, shared that he is 47 years old and never had a real job until this year (except selling drugs), proudly filing his first income tax return for 2018. On drugs for decades, incarcerated for 12 years, and in recovery for 3 years, his first job for the last 18 months has been with the Recovery Center, on the QRT. He vividly understands the life of addiction, but still lives in this local neighborhood. Some there don't recognize him, as he is 85 pounds heavier and got his teeth repaired. Obviously, he doesn't hang out with his old drug-using buddies.

Kenny says you have to tell folks the truth and that truth sometimes hurts. He relates that there are always excuses to get high, but that he now sees people with SUD as God sees them: broken, but with good stuff within. Kenny states, "If God loves you, I have to love you. He forgave—I forgive," and that, for their clients, he wants to "Love them to life, versus love them to death." When the team went in this past Monday, there were only eight overdoses, versus the 25-30 when he first started on the team.

The QRT does indeed work as a jazz ensemble. They wind up supporting people emotionally after deaths in their families and checking up on them after detox and treatment. One woman's mother had died, and she was back on drugs, but a visit from the team helped her get back to treatment and on to a clean lifestyle. The team sees their goal as helping people get clean and stay clean. They turn no one away. One woman was even driven to treatment in Baltimore. Happily, that woman is now 30 months clean, alive and functioning well.

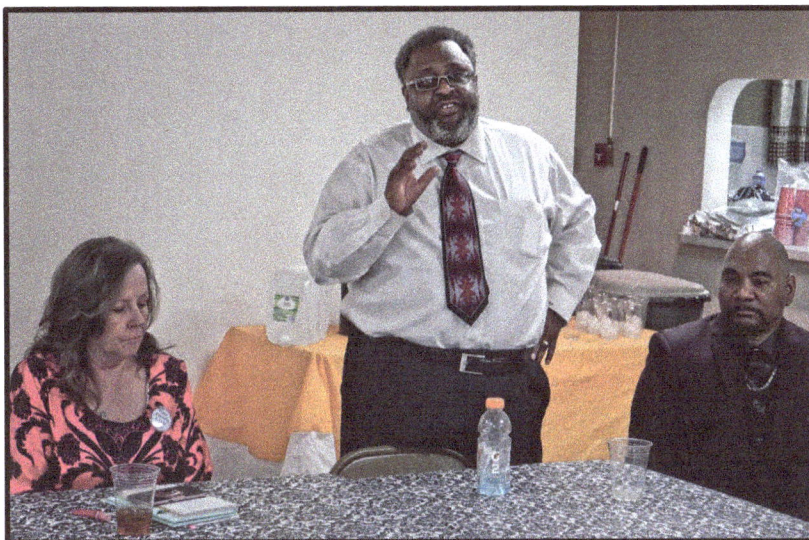

Terry Collison, Charles Shaw, Virgil Johnson

Ben, in his prior role on the police department, used to just throw everyone in jail for three days. He then realized that they needed a new tool, because jail stays didn't work. He sees how different people have different needs, and the diversity of the team helps with that. Pastor Virgil Johnson, one of the clergy team, can often pray over persons who are open to that, and it helps in a way that no other team members can. Some team members use humor to "reach" persons they visit, and that helps the team cope, too.

Bishop Shaw now only sets up schedules, but initially made visits too. He recalls a tough case of a young man they worked with in a local park, exemplifying "meeting them where they are." The mother was there with the son, and each of the team took turns, talking with the young man for over two hours. Finally, Larrecsa achieved a breakthrough when the young man admitted he was in pain from an infectious disease. She was able to talk him into going to the ED for treatment. The young man rode with his mother and Kenny to the ED. Bishop Shaw got in the car with Ben and sighed, saying, "Thank you, Jesus." Ben said, "Don't start that yet," and they all had a great laugh. Again, another success story is that this young man is clean and now doing well, which is quite rewarding.

When the faith leaders joined the team, the QRT didn't want them to judge or evangelize, just offer support. The QRT now sees how valuable that spiritual support is for those they visit, and to deal with the team's internal sorrow when someone dies. Pastor Duane Little came here from metro Detroit suburbs and his colleagues questioned his sanity in moving to Huntington, given the opioid epidemic. He has found that working on the QRT got him connected to "know and hear the street life and language." Being a part of the team opened his eyes, grounded him, and helped decrease his prior view of addiction: "That's just their choice."

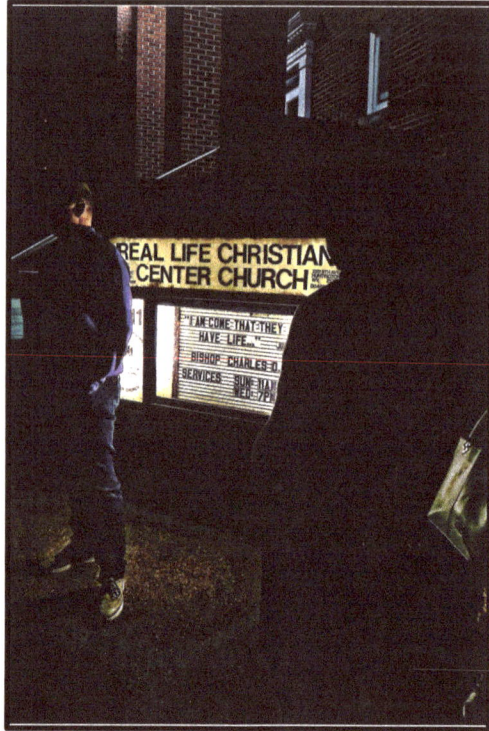

Real Life Christian Center Church

Now he understands the context and issues leading to and sustaining addiction and is helping to decrease that stigma. For him, he sees that each team member set aside their egos and go into the space where they can help best. Whoever connects best with the person goes in to help. In one case, a suicidal man in a hotel with his dog found out that Duane was a pastor and asked to talk. The rest of the team sat outside with the dog (but didn't bring this one home!).

Churches in general often exclude those who are addicted, wanting to stay within their four walls. Pastor Deb Winter's church in West End found out that every one of her members had been touched by drugs in the past 25 years. She asked them if they wanted to grow as a church and go into the ministry space of helping those with SUD. Some said yes and worked with her and some left. There was also another adjacent church parking lot where prostitution was taking place, so the need to refocus their ministry was evident.

They built a brand of recovery, and have a Celebrate Recovery service every Tuesday, with greater attendance than on Sunday morning. Their focus is on building relationships, "just like Jesus did". The original group of members had about 60 persons who left, but now 60 people regularly attend, particularly Celebrate Recovery.

Pastor Jamie Gump shared that there were many needles on the ground and members were angry that money was being spent on Narcan kits. Some people said, "Why not let them die?" Then an elderly person overdosed in his church. This changed a lot of attitudes toward opioid addiction. In 2002, fourteen young people died on Prom night, thanks to a drug deal that went bad. Overdoses kept increasing. Soon Pastor Darrell Buttram conducted the funeral service of a 19-year-old man who had been clean for a year, but did one "last hit" for his 19th birthday and died. The funeral director who contacted him said that all other area pastors refused to conduct the service. When he held the funeral service, the Pastor saw all sorts of youth he knew come trailing through.

He wanted to do something besides funerals to help, and QRT gave him that opportunity, particularly the chance to be part of that first point of contact and build right relationships. Many pastors are now developing new attitudes toward those with SUD and are taking that message to the pulpit to change their members. Pastor Virgil Johnson shared a similar story about his members thinking that QRT, needle exchange, and providing overdose reversal kits (particularly for multiple overdoses) are enabling more drug addiction. In talking with a member who strongly held this belief, the pastor said to the man, "If it were your son overdosing, wouldn't you want that kit available to save his life, even if it's the hundredth time?" The member began to rethink his position in light of that probing question. Virgil sees the clergy's role as providing awareness and education about SUD to their members.

Another pastor moved here from Lexington, KY and got the usual comments, wondering why he would come where so much trouble exists. He feels that many persons were called to the heart or epicenter of opioid overdoses, so that they could be part of the solution. In his view, God takes a problem and makes it work for the good. All the pastors commented that the bonds from this shared work are strong and help them overcome any theological differences.

The same is true for levelling the playing fields of race and money with regard to addiction. The QRT goes to mansions in the most affluent neighborhoods where overdoses occur, along with dark abandoned drug houses in the poorest zip codes, where people are lying around with spoons, other paraphernalia, and drugs. CNN often comes to town to do stories on Huntington's efforts and the team made a point to have the crews film across all neighborhoods, not just the poorest ones, to highlight that point.

Chaplain Doug Pendleton worked in healthcare for 25 years, often in trauma centers. Those seeking Dilaudid several decades ago were denigrated by medical staff, even then. Doug was lauded by his peers when he agreed to use similar negative labels to describe those with SUD, who said, "Now you are one of us." He has matured through this work to see that even those with SUD are children of God and should be loved.

Another pastor shared that the QRT work reminds him of his own son, in his 20's and the message, "There but for the grace of God go I." He recalls riding with a young man who was in and out of consciousness as they drove to treatment in Charleston the day after a 25-year-old female died of an overdose. He tells stories to convince his members to see the opioid crisis with fresh and not jaded eyes.

Lutheran Pastor Kevin Mackey shared that he has adopted his granddaughter due to his own daughter being addicted. His congregation knows that story, and he also puts QRT information in the church letter calendar. In QRT, they meet families with children when the parents are deep in the throes of addiction. He said one woman said, "I saw it coming and gave my children to someone else." So many grandparents and other family members are now raising these children that the State is over-whelmed with needs of the grandparents. Pastor Mackey added that rais-ing his granddaughter is both his greatest joy and challenge, since she is ten years old and he is in his 60's.

A final word for the night was that Huntington has resilience and has become a City of Solutions because its leaders were able put aside their egos and self-interest for the common good.

Cleveland, Ohio

7. Public Health, Health System and Community Partners Coalition, developing a CHNA, The Center for Health Affairs

https://www.neohospitals.org/

Contact: Terry Allan, MPH, Health Commissioner, Cuyahoga County Board of Health

2 Attendees, 1 male, 1 female; both White

We met with Terry Allan (Health Commissioner, Cuyahoga County Board of Health) and Kirstin Craciun, (Director, Community Outreach, The Center for Health Affairs), about Cuyahoga County's shared Community Health Needs Assessment (CHNA) and local collaborative efforts. Kirstin represents the regional Northeast Ohio hospital association in the CHNA process of Cuyahoga County.

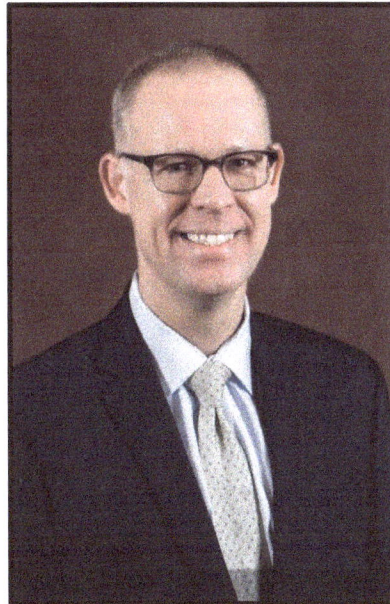

Terry explained that, with regard to the CHNA statutorily, Ohio is different from many other states. One factor is that the three major systems (Cleveland Clinic, Metro Health, University Hospital) are aligning their efforts with state requirements. When Kasich was the Governor, Greg Moody (Office of Health Transformation, State of Ohio) wanted to look at cost drivers for health. Moody brought together multi-sectoral stakeholders to push for three-year health assessments (versus five for health departments), to

Terry Allan

converge toward the health system IRS timeline. Health departments have State Health Improvement Plan (SHIP) requirements that call for a linkage to statewide priorities for health improvement. These efforts bridged healthcare and public health.

Ohio also expanded Medicaid, which resulted in almost 300,000 additional people covered, who received treatment and prevention services. A timeline was established statutorily (House Bill 390, 2016) so that all entities

Kirsten Craciun

would converge with the three-year community health assessment process.

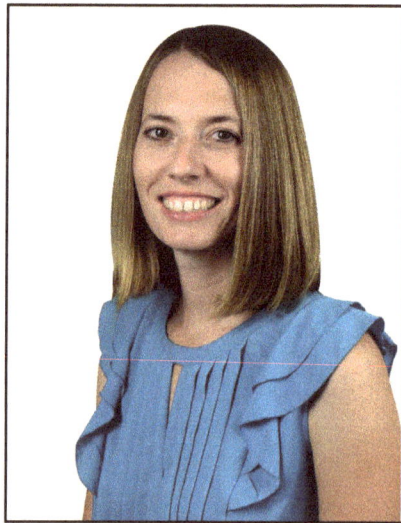

There was some dialogue about the concept of regional assessments; but that was seen as impractical and an effort to further consolidate local government, so it was not implemented. [Greg is now faculty at Ohio State's John Glenn College of Public Affairs.]

Four hospitals or systems (The MetroHealth System, Southwest General Health Center, St. Vincent Charity Medical Center, and University Hospitals) now work collaboratively with the two public health departments, Cuyahoga County Board of Health, and the Cleveland Department of Public Health, on their health assessments. The former plans created were independent and non-collaborative.

Kirstin was tasked with coordinating this collaborative CHNA with her co-chair, Dr. Heidi Gullett, from Case Western Reserve University's School of Medicine. The 2019 collaborative planning group included the Cuyahoga County Board of Health, the Cleveland Department of Public Health, MetroHealth, Southwest General Health Center, St. Vincent Charity Medical Center, and University Hospitals.

To realign the disparate hospital assessment cycles, they did a CHNA in 2018 *and* one in 2019, which was a huge undertaking. As a result, University Health moved from conducting eight assessments for each of their Cuyahoga County hospital facilities at the county level. Danielle Price (Director of Community Health Engagement), working under Heidi Gartland (Vice President of Government and Community Relations at University Health), was a champion in making this happen.

The heavy lift of getting all hospitals into alignment now has been accomplished. Cleveland Clinic (CC) has been at the table, but define their service area using zip codes, thus are precluded from participating in the county-level CHNA (which defines Cuyahoga County as the service area). Cleveland Clinic is still oriented to zip code level versus county, but is very interested in collaborating with the Cuyahoga County partners on implementing strategies to address shared health priorities.

The overarching themes that emerged from the dialogue in constructing the 2019 Cuyahoga County CHNA were structural racism, and trust. Five domains of top health needs included quality of life (poverty, homicide/violence/safety, food insecurity, and transportation), chronic disease (cardiovascular disease, childhood asthma, diabetes), health behaviors (flu vaccination rates, tobacco use, lack of physical activity), mental health and addiction (suicide, opioids/substance use disorders) and maternal/child health (infant mortality and lead poisoning).

Data sources included key stakeholder interviews, focus groups with social service providers, surveys mailed and administered by community health workers, public health and population level data, and hospital data.

To prioritize top areas of need, they asked these questions.

- How many people are affected? (magnitude)
- How likely is it to limit length and quality of life (severity)
- Does it impact some populations more than others? (inequity)
- How much of each population group is affected and are there differences? (magnitude of health disparity)
- How highly was health topic rated by community stakeholders and residents? (community priorities)
- Does it align with health priorities in the 2019 State Health Assessment? (alignment with the state).

Voting breakdown for further prioritization indicated that 20% of the votes reflected community voices, 40% represented hospitals, and 40% represented the city and county health departments.

The qualitative data from residents was very candid. Examples included comments such as: "Trust is a major issue. As a patient a person is stripped of their identify…." (pages 27-28). Having multiple partners involved in the CHNA offers a bit of diffusion of responsibility, as the community sentiments reflect the need for systemic change.

The final five selected health priorities were structural racism (intentional and unintentional racial bias across and within a society), trust, chronic disease (cardiovascular disease and diabetes), community conditions (homicides/violence/safety, poverty, transportation) and mental health and addiction (mental health/suicide, opioid/substance use disorders). For more details, see final CHNA report at 2019 Assessment [hipcuyahoga.org].

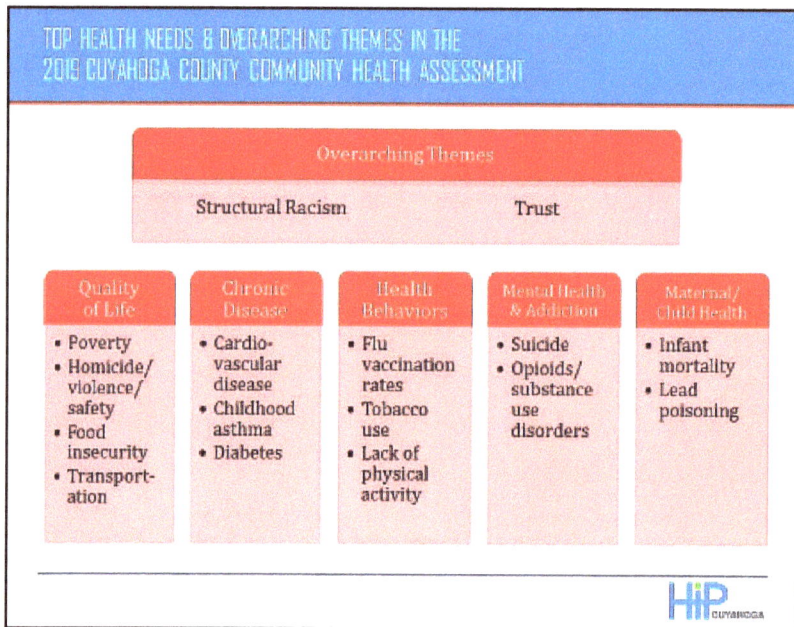

TOP HEALTH NEEDS & OVERARCHING THEMES IN THE 2019 CUYAHOGA COUNTY COMMUNITY HEALTH ASSESSMENT

Overarching Themes

Structural Racism   Trust

Quality of Life	Chronic Disease	Health Behaviors	Mental Health & Addiction	Maternal/ Child Health
• Poverty • Homicide/ violence/ safety • Food insecurity • Transport-ation	• Cardio-vascular disease • Childhood asthma • Diabetes	• Flu vaccination rates • Tobacco use • Lack of physical activity	• Suicide • Opioids/ substance use disorders	• Infant mortality • Lead poisoning

HiP CUYAHOGA

Cuyahoga County CHNA Themes

There is already work underway in Cuyahoga County to address structural racism and health disparities. A Forum on the "400 Years of Inequity" was recently held in Cleveland with attendees participating from multiple states in the Midwest. The Greater Cleveland health and social service community is now discussing racism openly, with agencies beginning to learn about the history of power and privilege, as well as changing their internal policies to expand job and contracting opportunities for people of color. There is a push on talking with African Americans and other patients of color who are mothers, and understanding perceptions of how their care is delivered in terms of intangibles factors (i.e., are they treated compassionately, with respect, etc., especially if on public assistance?). United Way of Greater Cleveland used the local CHNA as part of their gap analysis related to their Accountable Health Communities work. An alliance is coalescing in the community to more openly discuss and address racism, and the hope is that many other agencies will follow.

Locally, infant mortality rates are abysmal, with African American babies dying at much higher rates than White babies. In September 2019, a very powerful movie, *Toxic: A Black Woman's Story*, premiered in Cleveland. It describes a day in the life of an African American woman who is pregnant, and the myriad challenges she faces because of bias, power and privilege inequities in our community, and the toxic stress on moms and babies that is precipitated by these inequities.

Entities in Ohio are coordinating public health work and focusing on the doulas (trained professionals who provide continuous physical, emotional and informational support to a mother before, during and shortly after childbirth) doing the work on the ground to improve infant mortality rates, while looking at the possibility of Medicaid reimbursement and trying to keep funding directed there.

They are also meeting with local health systems, and public health and other stakeholders, to try to create a standard information system platform that could be shared. In fact, a local network of social service agency directors helped review the CHNA qualitative data and provided context for community concerns expressed in the listening sessions.

In Cleveland, in terms of trying to achieve improved community health outcomes, there is a shift toward foundations offering funding to social service agencies that address social determinants. For example, in Cleveland, "Say Yes to Education" is a national program (also similar efforts are underway in Buffalo, NY and Kalamazoo, MI). The program offers a long-term commitment to guarantee college tuition to every student who makes it through high school, up to $125M. Cleveland Foundation is the lead entity.

CHNA collaborative partners are creating a "to-do list" for the collaborative CHNA partners now that the findings are compiled. The momentum up to now has been to get systems aligned, but moving forward, the findings from the report must be addressed meaningfully. Case Western Reserve University's Center for Community Health Integration applied for a RWJF grant, which was successfully funded, to use community-based system dynamics to align partnerships, create a detailed understanding of how structural racism impacts in Cuyahoga County, and, most importantly, to identify actionable strategies to address structural racism at the system level. The partner organizations are hopeful that this funding will add momentum to the effort to work on a joint project.

Gary asked, "What could other states, like North Carolina, do to improve equity, based on the learning from Cleveland? In Ohio, the state mandated a move from five to three-year CHNA cycle (HB 390, passed in 2016) and offered $12K to each county to fund this effort for one year. That helped nominally to move the work forward. However, the true question is what to do with current CHNA findings. That is the big task before the Cleveland and Cuyahoga County teams now.

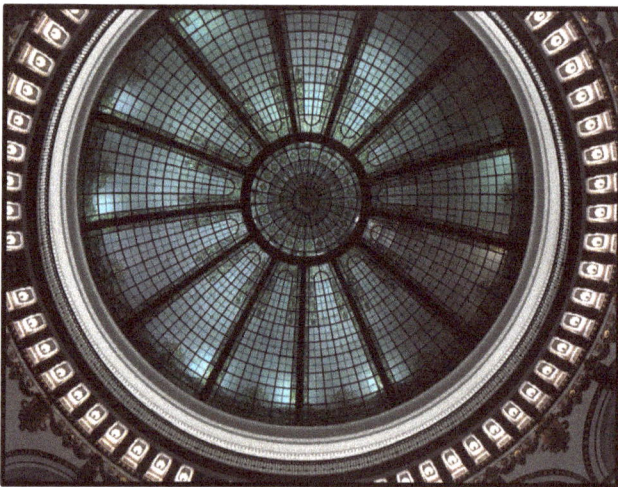

Cleveland, Ohio

8. University Hospitals, Rainbow Babies & Children's Hospital

https://www.uhhospitals.org/rainbow

Contacts: Heidi Gartland; VP, Government & Community Relations, University Hospitals; Laura Chiarelli, Danielle Price, Director of Community Engagement

5 Attendees, 2 male, 3 female; 4 White, 1 AA

We met with Tom Zenty, CEO, University Hospitals, Dan Simon, MD, Chief Clinical & Scientific Officer of University Hospitals & President, UH Cleveland Medical Center, and Heidi Gartland, Vice President of Government and Community Relations for University Hospitals about health system and community partnerships. We continued our conversation over lunch with Heidi Gartland, Patti DePompei, RN, President of Rainbow Babies & Children's and MacDonald Women's hospitals, and Danielle Price, Director, Community Health Engagement for University Hospitals.

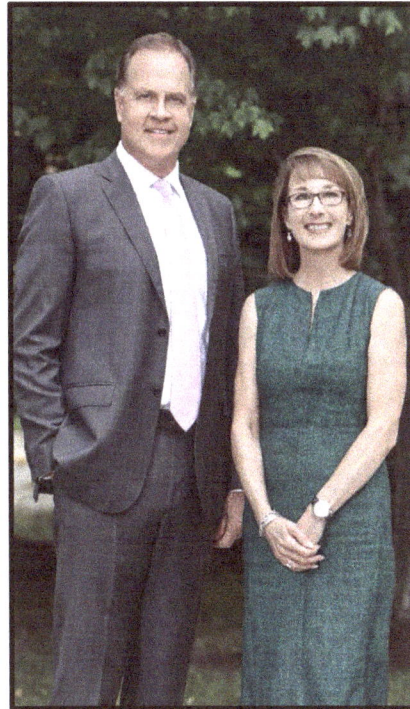

Tom Zenty and Heidi Gartland

Many of Cleveland's leaders of business, religion and medicine came together in May of 1866, pledging to build a hospital where "the most needy would be considered the most worthy." Community

Benefit for FY18 was $383M. Some programs are very innovative. Vision 2010 was a campus transformation project ($1.2B) that focused on driving positive change in the community by utilizing local construction companies and vendors owned by minorities and women. In the last 10 years, about $785M dollars went to these groups. At that time, it was very novel and opened doors for minority and women-owned businesses in the city.

Fundamentally, its leadership knows that structural racism and poverty are closely associated so they strive to be an inclusive organization. At the Anchor Institution meeting, that was a key point. When they conducted the CHNA in Cuyahoga County, the data revealed that they have roughly 5 times the Ohio state average for mortality rates for infants born to AA mothers: 15.6/1000 for African American babies in Ohio vs. 3.76/1000 for Caucasian babies in Cuyahoga County.

In general, African American babies die at a rate three times that of white babies in Ohio and roughly four times the rate in Cuyahoga County. Research shows that 80% of the factors that determine our health are not related to the medical care received but rather the impact on bodies from environmental, behavioral and socioeconomic factors. And while we are an advanced nation, considerable disparities exist in health care.

UH is committed to improving the health of the communities they serve. It took an affirming step in 2018 to close the health care disparity gap by opening the UH Rainbow Center for Women & Children. UH convened a community advisory group around the Hough neighborhood (3 miles from the main campus), where residents' lifespan is 24 years shorter in mortality compared to a nearby middle class suburb. They developed a program and put up a building to address perinatal and prenatal pregnancy issues via a model of Centering Pregnancy.

UH has the largest Centering Pregnancy regional model in Ohio. That program started in 2010, after midwives approached Patti about no-show rates and wanted to know how UH could help. Ohio State Medicaid recognizes the great outcomes, breastfeeding, better infant health, etc., achieved by Centering Pregnancy compared to traditional medical care. The program addresses diet, nutrition, cooking and general pediatrics. The Rainbow Center includes acute walk-ins, and is strategically located near two bus stops. It offers onsite dental, vision, optometry, legal navigation (e.g. eviction), utility assistance, WIC office, an onsite pharmacy with 340B, which permits meds to beds for the hospital, behavioral health, and food access. They were able to negotiate having a partner place a 50,000 square foot grocery store across the street. It contains a test kitchen, where staff teach folks to shop for, prepare and cook healthy food.

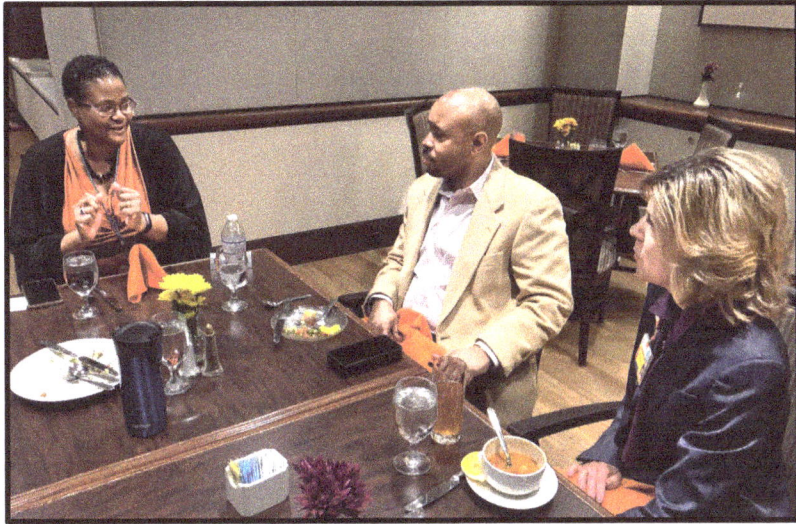

Danielle Price, Jeremy Moseley, Patti DePompei

UH leadership saw the investment as a social responsibility requirement; the great news is they didn't do it alone. Many generous donors stepped forward to make their mark in helping improve the overall health and wellness of the Cleveland community. Since opening nearly two years ago, the Center has provided nearly 130,000 clinical care and pharmacy visits. Since the Centering Program began in 2010, helped by the initiative at the UH Rainbow Center for Women & Children, pre-term birth rates declined from 8% in 2010 to just 6% in 2019 and low birth rate babies have decreased from 8% to 7%.

Clearly, as UH moves to Population Health, this kind of care model will help them shift from fee-for-service to value-based payments. A very early benefit they have seen, indirectly, because UH put in an acute care walk-in clinic at the new Rainbow Center, is that 2,000 pediatric cases have been diverted from the ED.

How do the providers see this? They have embraced it completely. The General Internal Medical group loves it. Obstetrics care is much improved. The environment is very pleasant, and they are now renovating the ED for specialty care (e.g., Nephrology, Neurology) with some of the "savings" from this diversion. This has also spun redevelopment in the area. There was one for-profit before, but their building helps; housing is getting better. Jobs and businesses are moving into the area. In their UH careers Tom (17 yrs) and Dan (14 yrs) have worked a lot on fundraising; tons of leadership time is devoted to this. People are requesting that they create a similar Rainbow Center in other places, with higher rates of African American and Hispanic populations.

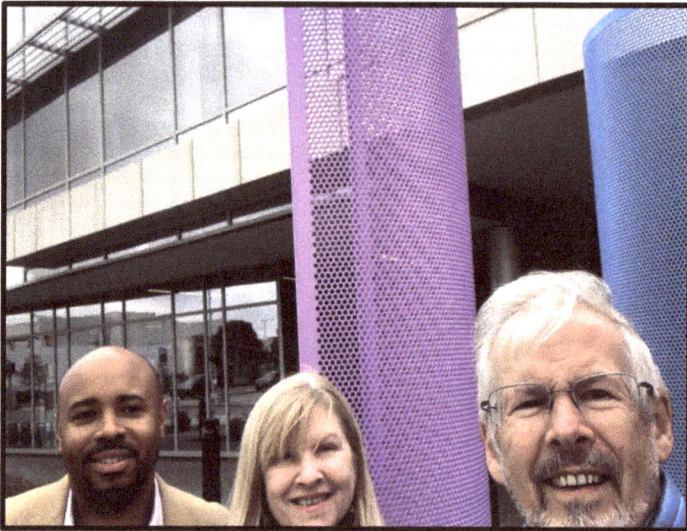

Jeremy Moseley, Teresa Cutts and Gary Gunderson at the Rainbow Center

Patti DePompei shared with us more details about the Rainbow Center's success at lunch. She said that her fundraising efforts for the Rainbow Center were so special. Presenting the data and showing what UH wanted to do to change was amazing and helped with fundraising. Initially, building the Center was a leap of faith. They did a lot of advance analysis. Patti started in 2012; she wanted to deliver Primary Care differently. The clinic that was close by was not ideal and parking was difficult. UH identified the existing users to learn more about what might work.

Theirs was a truly participative effort with the local community, down to the design and decoration of the Center. They developed a

Community Advisory Board (CAB) and made no assumptions about colors or design. The users' opinions, including faith community representatives, juveniles, other health care providers too, mattered more. The art was selected by the CAB. Everyone invited came to the meeting. UH discovered that relationship building is key, which signaled to the community that their input is important.

Fundraising came from the Development office. They got the CAB involved and they became large contributors of ideas, secondary to data and stories. The Center was built on a vacant lot, with little around it. Now there are more stores and a grocery store across the street.

Once the Rainbow Center opened, it was clear that men in the neighborhood needed a similar focus on their health. The UH Otis Moss Jr. Health Center was identified as the solution. Located down the street in the Fairfax neighborhood, this Center was expanded to provide a Food for Life Market, which has provided more than 740 individuals with free healthy food options since it opened in 2018.

Working with the Cleveland Food Bank and Sodexo, patients can get a food referral that is good for six months. If further assistance is needed the patient can come back to see their primary care physician for another referral. The Food For Life Market now serves 13 different communities. UH provides space, and Sodexo provides the Registered Dietitian to educate and guide their patients as they shop through the market.

And in March 2020, the Otis Moss Center announced the opening of a Brain Health Clinic, on-demand access to non-urgent care, a new diagnostic radiology suite, and workforce development programs. This reinvigorated Center cares for people with chronic illness, cognitive and behavioral health issues.

UH also offers a unique service: bedside voting on Election Day if a county resident is in the hospital. If kids are in the hospital, the parents can vote, too; this required a law change. The county sends voting registration representatives to help with this effort.

Danielle Price, Director of Community Health Engagement, was asked how they managed to commit to reducing structural racism, which often occurs across the country, not just in Cuyahoga County, and grow trust in the CHNA in these tough times. There was fertile ground upon which to build this. In 2013, the county first declared reducing structural racism as a priority. Other stakeholders have come in (Racial Equity Institute) to build the capacity of local leaders.

Particularly in the infant mortality space for African-American women, there is a need to name it and address it, as it has been taboo for so long. All the unconscious bias around it is also an issue. First Year Cleveland is an infant mortality initiative and Patti and Heidi keep the space clear for that work to proceed at UH.

The Center for Health Affairs has been instrumental in getting Cuyahoga County stakeholders to cooperate in a collaborative county level CHNA. The steering committee meets once a month. The process also happens in the other 5 counties where UH hospitals are located; most of the rural counties have been collaborating a long time. Cuyahoga has so many resources that here it's more of an issue of co-ordinating, aligning, and not stepping on toes of partners.

A convener is needed to manage the process and the Center for Health Affairs takes on this role, as one of the oldest ones in the country. In addition to the city and county public health departments, UH, St. Vincent Charity, Southwest General, and Metro Health are involved. Now, they are trying to go into a space to keep the collaboration alive and dynamic and useful, with shared implementation and projects.

Danielle worked previously at Neighborhood Connections, managing the community engagement process for the Greater University Circle (GUC) anchor strategy. GUC is nationally recognized for the Evergreen Cooperatives. She was part of a collaborative team trying to identify mutually beneficial opportunities for the grasstops and grassroots.

Through Neighborhood Connections, a program of the Cleveland Foundation, over 200 grassroots groups per year receive up to $5K to implement projects to improve the quality of life in their neighborhood. Neighborhood Connects played an integral role in connecting diverse groups of people by creating easy on-ramps for relationship building. It's an ongoing process to give voice to all. Danielle sees that the level of door-knocking you have to do in community, you also have to do inside the hospital.

Illuminating issues through data and stories is one of the most important things they do to engage community and others. Patti gave the example of how they used to share data points about the safety concerns of neglecting hand-washing, but it paled in comparison to displaying a photo of nine babies to represent the number of causalities that occur based on infections associated with germs on the provider's hands. That worked in changing behavior for better outcomes.

Likewise, Danielle talked about early successes regarding the use of a move to make sure that providers and the community really understand the underlying causes of disparities related to infant mortality. *Toxic: A Black Woman's Story* is a movie about a day-in-the-life of a pregnant AA woman, which will be broadly distributed to the public soon.

9. Evergreen Cooperatives

http://www.evgoh.com/about-us/

Contact: John McMicken, CEO,
Evergreen Cooperative, Green City Growers

Attendee: 1 white male

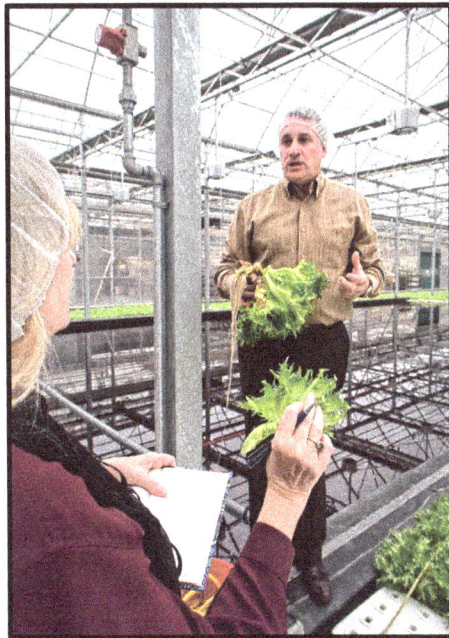

Teresa Cutts and John McMicken

Launched in 2008 by a working group of Cleveland-based institutions (including the Cleveland Foundation, the Cleveland Clinic, University Hospitals, Case Western Reserve University, and the municipal government), the Evergreen Co-operative Initiative is working to create living-wage jobs, this in six low-income neighborhoods with a median household income below $18,500, in an area known as Greater

University Circle. We met with its CEO, John McMicken, at their Green City Growers site, one of four ventures (which also includes Evergreen Cooperative Laundry, Evergreen Energy Solutions, and Evergreen Business Services). Evergreen Cooperatives is a 10% not-for-profit and 90% employee-owned model.

Evergreen Cooperatives' website states that it:

"... was designed to create an economic breakthrough in Cleveland. Rather than a trickle-down strategy, it focuses on economic inclusion and building a local economy from the ground up. Rather than offering public subsidy to induce corporations to bring what are often low-wage jobs into the city, the Evergreen strategy calls for catalyzing new businesses, owned by their employees. Rather than concentrate on workforce training for employment opportunities that are largely unavailable to low-skill and low-income workers, the Evergreen Initiative first creates the jobs, and then recruits and trains local residents to fill them.

The Evergreen Cooperative Initiative remains an important model for healing neglected post-industrial economies in the American heartland. But it's also part of a larger initiative in alternative wealth-building and wealth-sharing models being considered by stakeholders in the Greater University Circle Initiative. Says the Cleveland Foundation's President/CEO and Evergreen Board Chairman, Ronn Richard: "Our goal is equitable wealth creation at scale."

John shared some general information about Evergreen Cooperatives and then walked us through the Green City Growers site, offering particular details on that arm of the Co-op. One of the early challenges was building the initiative to large enough scale. Early feasibility studies about starting a laundry and hydroponic greenhouse suggested that stakeholders have to be truly a part of building a new business (not just donate money, pose for a photo opportunity, and go away), and that they had to create real jobs that generated enough income to make payroll. A leader was needed to make the Cooperative work and John stepped up from a former business background to fill that role.

The overall Co-op now has 225 employee owners with 55% of them formerly incarcerated. Interestingly, their turnover rate is lower than traditional businesses. Forty-two persons work at Green City Growers. They have two laundry sites, a solar panel construction site, and a business service that offers human resources, sales, accounting, and marketing. Co-ops are for-profit, but essentially tax neutral, as profits are redistributed to employees. Co-ops pass tax liability through to its employee owners. Their model is 25% profit (redistributed as a bonus) and 75% patronage account (like retirement income). Employees purchase one share at a cost of $3,000; this amount was designed to be affordable and financed through payroll deduction. Only one share can be purchased. The patronage account can be accessed immediately, usually by borrowing against it or using it as collateral. When an owner leaves, he/she gets a full refund; however, the company has up to five years to pay it out. Thus far, the Co-Op has

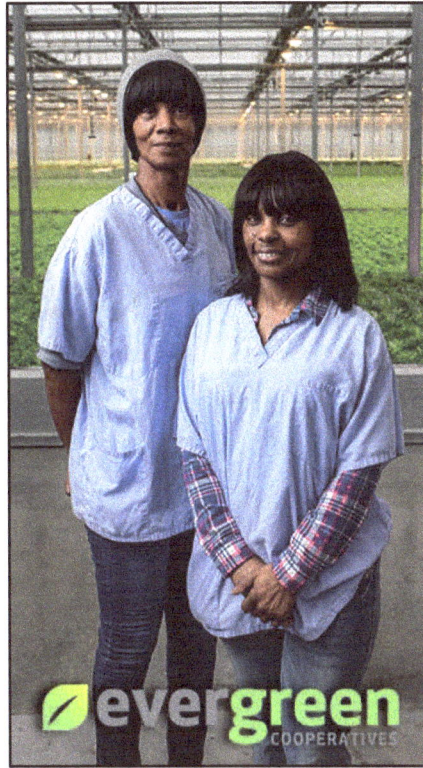

Evergreen Employee Owners Videllia Coleman & Shirley Gaston

always paid the patronage fee out immediately when an employee leaves, but a 5-year clause protects the company if numerous owners were to depart at the same time.

For the Green City Growers, the stars and factors aligned among the two hospitals, owners, community residents, the City of Cleveland, and Case Western to make this venture materialize. The communities themselves had created the poverty map of the areas, but Evergreen had to engage local residents in placing the facility in their neighborhood early on in the process. This built excitement and increased the level of collaboration among local residents, particularly since the Co-op had an impact on property values. Formerly there were 40 residences on the property and 37 of those were deemed blighted by the City. So, at the onset, there were opportunities for physical revitalization of neighborhoods and wealth creation by hiring local workers/employees. The Co-op aimed to replace the blight with tax-paying businesses in the area.

During start-up, Green City Growers required much more capital funding than they anticipated to build out services and make payroll. They had to learn how to alter, monitor and stabilize temperature as well as water quality inside the greenhouse, even during frigid Ohio winters. Artificial LED lighting is now used to complement sunlight.

They had difficulty initially getting a bank loan to cover the LED costs, but decreased their electric bill by 40% with this lighting change. They

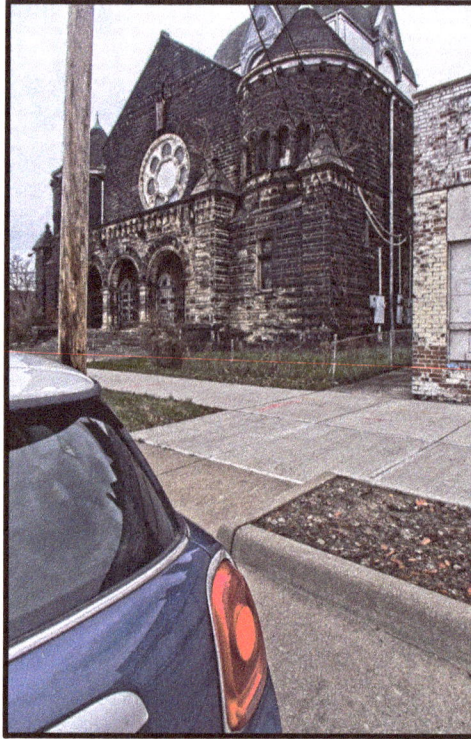

Cleveland Church near Evergreen Cooperative

use one million gallons of water per month for operations, but recycle rainwater, which requires no water from the local water treatment facility. As John puts it, "If the water is good, the plants are good." New job roles were created for technicians and mechanics to repair equipment for keeping temperature, humidity and water on track.

Their site is the size of 13 football fields with that many ponds, where they grow lettuce and herbs. Crops are rotated from one end to another; mature crops are moved and harvested at the end of the 45-day growing cycle. Employees and others have helped Green City Growers create their signature lettuce brands: Bouquet Blend (with six different lettuces), a variety out of the Netherlands with green leaf, iceberg, and a Romaine called Cleveland Crisp. They have had difficulty getting organic certification for hydroponic gardens as there is no soil involved, just purified rainwater, salt and other nutrients.

Ensuring a firm commitment from buyers for a product can mitigate risk. Even in Cleveland, only 30% of their product is bought by the hospitals' food distributors. As the quality of their products have gained recognition, they now provide to local restaurants, schools and grocery stores. Happily, too, Nestlé has their research and development lab (where recipe testing and food processing occurs) in Cleveland, and they buy about 30% of the fresh basil that Green City Growers produces, to insure good quality and availability of that product (roughly 4,000 pounds of basil per week). Green City Growers does not deliver product but does store it for buyers. In terms of the future of food, there is a need for food grown at a high level of safety, in a highly controlled environment, and where you need it (to curb the carbon footprint and insure freshness).

Laundry services have a huge spread and, if a company offers quality, they can make a profit. A few other cities have similar laundry models, like in West Chicago, where one site has a 75,000 square foot pilot employing 200 people, and is energy efficient. Now, highly technical maintenance of complex laundry facilities is a new type of job that is emerging and laundries are employee friendly—no longer sweatshops. Transportation for laundry is another aspect of the business that attracts many social entrepreneurs, as is linen and textile repair. They have recently created Evergreen University to teach others to build and sustain these types of businesses.

John shared some lessons learned. There have been some human resource challenges in using the employee owner model, particularly how to respect employees but still expect accountability and even terminate them at times. In terms of funding, philanthropy helped keep the business afloat. As mentioned before, they initially seriously under-capitalized their startup costs, so had to rely on donor monies to keep them operational in the first few years. John thinks having funding for at least three years, but up to five for more complex operations (like the greenhouse), for a start-up is ideal. Educating restaurants and other consumers on why their product costs 20% more than commercially grown brands has been difficult, though it helps that their product is higher quality, better tasting, and longer lasting than others.

Another area where Evergreen is leading innovation is in dealing with the "silver tsunami," as business owners exit a long-owned business. They lend money to help existing employees acquire an older company when an owner wants to retire. They have seen how these business closings can put their supply chain at risk. So, they are looking to convert these businesses to the employee owner model.

10. Cleveland Clinic, Pastoral Care and ACPE

https://my.clevelandclinic.org/departments/patient-experience/depts/
spiritual-care[my.clevelandclinic.org]

Contact: Rev. Dr. Amy Greene, Director of Spiritual Care

1 Attendees, 1 white female

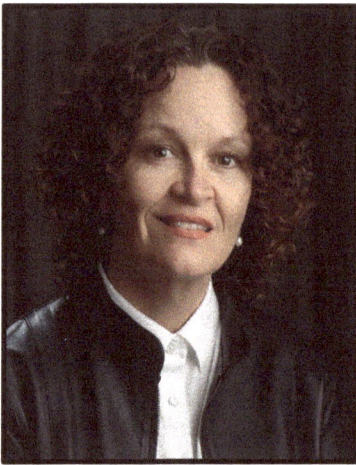

Amy Greene Dayton, Ohio

We discussed health system and chaplaincy efforts, especially in light of Rev. Dr. Amy Greene's current role as Board Chair of the Association for Clinical Pastoral Education (ACPE). Amy has been at Cleveland Clinic (CC) for 12 years. Hers is a small staff, including herself and six full-time chaplains, along with three ACPE educators and one candidate. Happily, she has a Rabbi and Muslim chaplain on staff now. Her CPE program has 12 Interns (basic unit) and 2 Residents (paid for the second year).

There are few good seminaries in Ohio, so a national search to recruit residents was needed. Recruiting from afar is not difficult, though, as Cleveland Clinic offers truly extraordinary learning opportunities for her chaplain residents and trainees. She is hopeful about using virtual visits going forward, for extended coverage with relatively few staff and a mandate from the new CEO, Dr. Tomislav "Tom" Mihaljevic, who started in 2017, to double the number of patients seen by the Clinic within the next 5 years.

Her team has been helping with Employee self-care after the death of a well-known patient who was seen by more than 500 providers here at CC over a period of 6 years. Amy is a certified teacher of Cognitively Based Compassion Training (out of Emory University's Tibetan Partnership) and conducts various mindfulness and meditation courses throughout the year.

Former CEO Dr. Toby Cosgrove was a huge force in getting CC on the international map. He is now starting up Cleveland Clinic, London. Dr. Adam Myers, from Texas, is the new head of Population Health and making different and interesting choices here at Cleveland in that domain. Amy would like to see Spiritual Care integrated into community outreach.

Amy is finishing her two-year term as Chair of the Board of the Directors of the Association for Clinical Pastoral Education, Inc. (ACPE). Leading ACPE with the constant change that seems to be part of modern healthcare has been a challenge, but Amy is excited about the groundwork that she helped to lay for more substantial partnerships—perhaps even a merger—with other major organizations for Spiritual Care and Educations, such as the Association of Professional Chaplains, the National Association of Catholic Chaplains, and Neshama, the Association for Jewish Chaplains. These groups and more will gather in Cleveland in May 2020 for a large summit.

The FaithHealth team from Wake Forest had already shared in 2016 about the Memphis Model and NC Way work with Amy and her local teams and faith community leaders. We were eager to hear what has grown out of those meetings. Unfortunately, there hasn't been much movement on the partnership, as there is too much to do inside the house, just serving 1400 beds and thousands of employees at the main campus. Additionally, three of the nine "smaller" regional hospitals in the northeast Ohio area have an average of 500 beds each. Her staff is extremely busy, but each of the other hospitals have at least one chaplain now.

Amy and her team are committed to Cleveland Clinic and the work that they have been doing here for over a decade.

Thursday, Nov. 21, 2019

Dayton, Ohio

11. Kettering Health System. Safety Net and Faith Community Partnerships, Grandview Hospital, Kettering

https://www.ketteringhealth.org/grandview/

Contact: Dr. Peter Bath, VP KHN Missions and Ministry, Kettering Health Network

24 Attendees, 12 male,12 female; 20 White,3 AA, I Hispanic

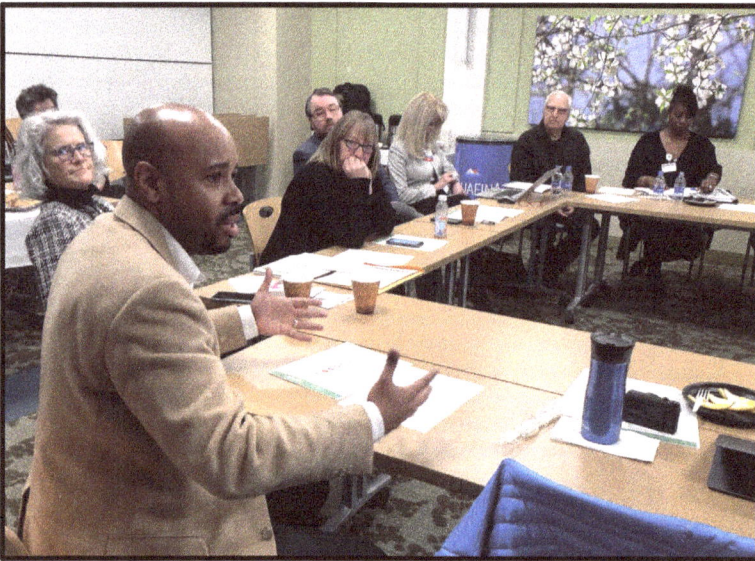

Jeremy Moseley, Kelly Fackel, Becky Lewis, Jill Kingston, PJ Brafford, Kathy Perno, Frank Perez, Lisa Anne Powe

We met with over 25 local leaders who shared about Kettering Health Network (KHN) and community and faith-based partnerships in the Dayton area. The group introduced themselves and their roles, and Peter Bath, VP KHN Missions and Ministry, offered a reflection about becoming "Other-Centric" and serving. P.J. Brafford, Network Government Relations Officer, offered a focus for this meeting: to listen carefully in a spirit of openness and thought-fulness. Health systems are crossing the sidewalk to learn the humble arts of supporting the community vital to health. Gary Gunderson (Secretary, Stakeholder Health and Wake Forest Baptist Health VP of FaithHealth) spoke about Stakeholder Health and the See2See tour.

P.J. Brafford shared that, while community benefit work is fundamentally driven by checking boxes for the IRS to protect our not-for-profit status, KHN is doing so much more in terms of building and supporting intentional partnerships in the community.

One supported program, Brigid's Path, was begun by its Executive Director, Jill Kingston, that focuses on the "God Moments." The program name came from Jill's spiritual background, Catholicism, referencing St. Brigid, the patron saint of newborns, and the Bible verse, Psalm 25: "Show me your ways, Lord and teach me your paths." However, the program itself is interfaith.

Jill and her husband started fostering drug-exposed babies and were ill-prepared to care for them. They have three biological children, plus two who were withdrawing from heroin. She was seeing what the hospitals were doing and the families' suffering, so felt a calling to do more and started researching what resources were available. She went to visit Mary at Lilly's Place in Huntington, West VA, as that group was about to start the first neonatal recovery system.

One example of "God's moments" was the story of how they found their building site. Brigid's Path had looked at many sites but, one day, stopped at a different site than what they planned. Jill's friend, who is a realtor, called and said that a family wanted to donate that building. Many architects and others stepped up to donate services (cost was $2M versus an estimated $4M). The building had to be gutted. Usually $60-80K to do this, they had 100 people show up to volunteer to gut it. A well-dressed lady arrived (not prepared for renovation work) who said that she was praying and God told her to come. She shared that she had just met someone who, after a quick call from this lady, provided three new dumpsters within 30 minutes to contain the debris generated from gutting the building. Brigid's Path also got their 501c3 expedited, while the community surrounded them with gifts of diapers, architects, and many other people and resources. They had to change zoning locally and licensing paths, since the program's work was brand new. Experts stepped up to help.

Brigid's Path is a home-like setting that offers care 24 hours/7 days a week from skilled medical staff and volunteers. Many Moms are frightened and need to be loved and cared for in this critical time. In the hospital, the babies are scored in terms of acuity of symptoms, and many of them drop 5 points immediately upon entering the space, because of the relaxed atmosphere. They aim to try to care for the babies without drugs. Babies can stay up to 90 days and Moms can room in as well.

Since December 2017 Brigid's Path has cared for 63 babies and some Moms. They provide hope and help for the Mom, as well as for families (who often are estranged). They meet the Mom "wherever" she is to provide support.

One Mom with a brain tumor, on the medication Neurontin, needed extra support and she and her baby received care. They have 135 trained cuddlers who tend to the babies. Cuddlers have shots and background checks and training to learn about the babies' needs, and how to be trauma-informed and sensitive with the Moms and families. They help with laundry and front desk needs as well. Brigid's Path has had 1600 applications to volunteer.

Jill's dream is to assign mentors to each Mom. The mentors could give Mom a ride, provide diapers, whatever she might need. Transportation and housing are big needs. After discharge, Moms often go back to unhealthy settings and situations. House Bill 115 is creating amazing support for Moms who are in addiction. Jill's background is in education and she says that "God is qualifying me." She noted the many different languages, acronyms, etc. that she has had to learn in this work. PJ has been a blessing to her and the team in this learning journey and is on their Board.

Bev Knapp (VP of Clinical Integration and Innovation) is the voice helping Kettering remember the heart of the mission. Despite the technical language of check boxes and acronyms (Community Health Needs Assessment or CHNA), community benefit serves "our churches, corporations, our first responders and at-risk populations," all of whom have varied needs. It's hard work to care for those who might avoid screening for cancer, for example. They are a resource and provide education, screen, equip audiences with skills, and provide the ability to expand capacity. They like to see Population Health outcomes change but note that this is hard to track accurately in community.

CHNA priorities include Mental Health/Substance Abuse (MH/SA), access to care, Chronic Disease, and Healthy Behavior.

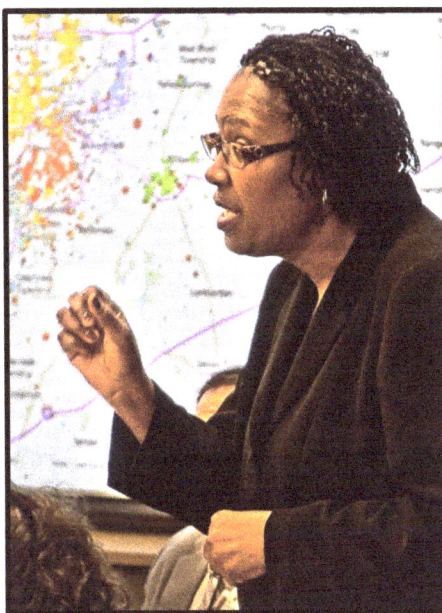

Karen Young, Dayton Scholars

Partners in this work include the Good Neighbor House, Infant Mortality Task Force, and the Hope Center for Families, along with Brigid's Path and dozens of others. They are screening pastors and spouses to promote health and to engage congregations, and have offerings in terms of rural health, midwifery, and prenatal care. The Congregational Health Model was just approved by the Board and is now beginning.

Val Parker Haley shared that they have 103 resourced staff, including registered nurses, nurse practitioners, massage therapists, dieticians and non-clinical staff that offer services. They have a call center for coordinating these services. Lisa Ann Powe shared about their Creation Health program, slated to start in 2020.

Community Outreach put this together: "Ten Weeks to CREATION" Health (Choice, Rest, Environment, Activity, Trust, Interpersonal Relationships, Outlook, Nutrition). Participants start class with baseline measurements of weight and other vitals and bring a buddy. After the 10th class, participants repeat baseline biometrics. Participants move from episodic data to a long-term cohort to demonstrate impact. Congregations are natural places for this to happen.

Greater Allen AME Church is a place where similar work has occurred. Bonnie Baker Tattershall (Community Engagement Manager, KHN) shared that, of the 400 congregants at their church, most have been touched by the program. The pastor credits a men's health seminar last year with saving his life. If the Pastor and First Lady are healthy, that trickles down positively through the whole congregation. Free mammography has been offered via the Grandview Foundation. Greater Allen AME says that many members have been inspired to obtain more mammograms via this program, after many years of not having access. Bonnie serves as the interfaith outreach coordinator with the congregations.

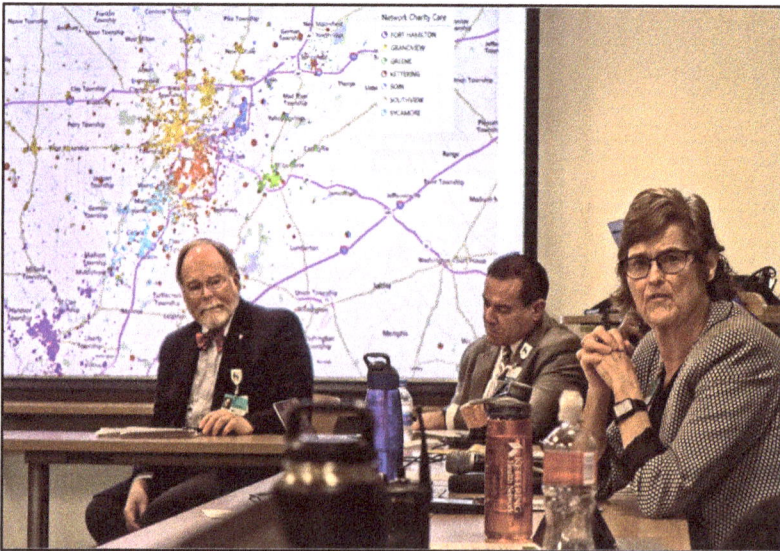

Peter Bath, Bill Largo, Bev Knapp

Kettering Health Network (KHN), a seven-hospital system, mapped the hotspots of I-75. For Grandview, the hotspots of 160,000 persons are closest to the inner-city. The Good Neighbor House and Primary Health Solutions are located in the epicenter of these high utilizers. They stop the need by helping them get care sooner rather than later; not by saying "No" to providing care. They want people to learn how to move care upstream. Community benefit, in the past, used to be what was offered if you had a successful year in terms of margin. Now, in the risk-based contract world, community benefit can be the leading edge, not the trailing edge. Great, robust community partners are a critical part of their health system strategy. KHN now has 75,000 lives in their Clinically Integrated Network; 14,000 are Medicaid patients and they struggle with volume, ED visits and doing the right thing for patients. The Stakeholder group shared about the collaborative CHNA in Cleveland, with the top two priorities addressing structural racism and trust.

In the Dayton area, the Greater Dayton Area Hospital Association or GDAHA (with many counties with different ways of measuring) just completed their 3rd iteration of the collaborative CHNA. Reducing heart attack mortality and other goals are being set as top priorities. Focusing on zip code and census tract or even streets, targeting outcomes, is helpful. Bev plans to do that at population and congregational level here. In Tampa, they found a hotspot area and brought a clinic into that space.

Primary Health Solutions, the new local FQHC that is partnering with Kettering, offers a unique delivery model. Mark Bellisario (President) and Steven Roller (CMO) offered descriptions of this model. Their job is not to judge, but to meet people where they are. They added a focus on goals of decreasing infant mortality and improving behavioral health. They work with the school-based health center as they believe that all roads lead to the children and early development. If kids miss school because of asthma or behavioral health reasons, that causes problems later on, including lower employment opportunities. Helping the families earlier improves self-esteem and helps with employment (dental care helps, particularly, in this regard too). Starting early with providing help is important. They wrap all those services in one building and screen everyone for alcohol, drugs, and depression. Steve wants to integrate behavioral health in their primary care setting.

Transportation is a huge barrier. Their clinics are on a bus route, but they try to provide as many outpatient services in one location for convenience. Even in terms of electronic health records (EHR), the primary care provider can make this a barrier. Now all services are on the same EHR and they are seeing better outcomes for patients.

The partnership with KHN has been a blessing. In the past, it was frustrating for FQHCs because they were in a "one-down" position with respect to health systems. Now the healthcare world is changing, and they are hopeful that in the current reimbursement model these partnerships can work for the good of all. Primary Health Solutions is primarily based in Butler County. Its leaders began to talk with KHN leaders when Good Samaritan Hospital in West Dayton was closing. There were already two FQHCs in Dayton, but there was still a huge, unmet need in this area. As they planned the new center, they hired a pediatrician, because the community members said they needed that. They were already in a partnership with North Ridge when a tornado came through and caused more damage and increased that need.

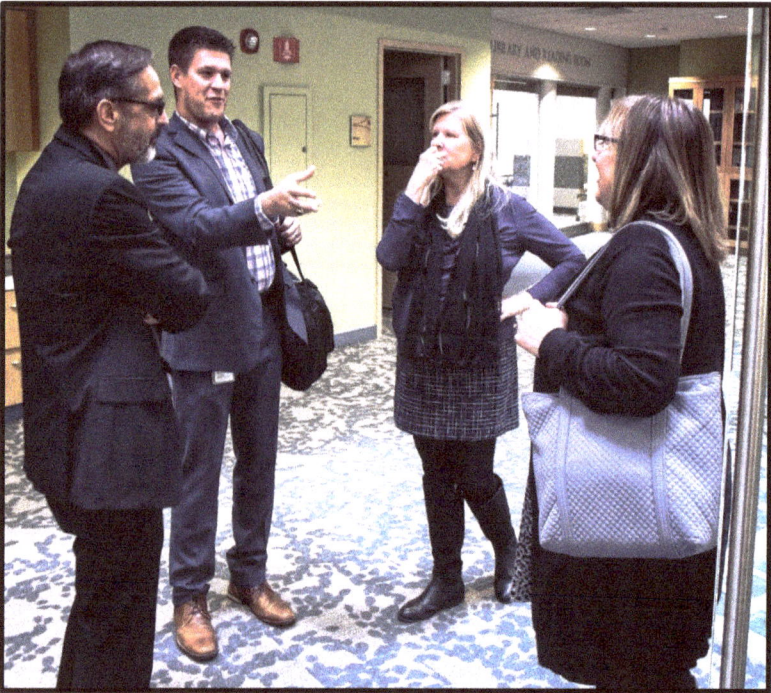

Marc Bellisario, Steven Roller, Teresa Cutts, Jill Kingston

As an FQHC, they can now pay for psychiatry. From school-based systems alone they made over 800 referrals for behavioral health last year. They have certified application counselors for Medicaid. They try to identify barriers and overcome them. In Butler County, as part of the infant mortality initiative, they offer wellness visits, safety assessment, and WIC connections—over 700 visits for these services last year. Patients really appreciate their one stop shop and care.

They are adding a fourth partnership with the school-based centers, which run year-round (to create a medical home). They get parents' consent to treat (vision, dental, medical, hearing on site). Amazingly, the county made the consent form good through 12th grade and the consent form travels with the child, as the families are often very mobile. The school bought a van and provide a transporter. They bring kids to the school-based health center, so parents don't lose time from work.

PJ notes that there is a move toward putting a human face on the logistical details and form-signing backdoor operations that can make the health system and other stakeholder partnerships more successful. The partnerships seem more horizontal, in that partners bring a lot to the table. Bev recognizes that "co-opetition" is key; KHN needs to provide better management to 'their' Medicaid patients, and partnerships like those with Primary Health Solutions are especially critical. The value to the community and providers is also important. Ten percent of FQHC's patients are commercially insured, so it's not just care for the poor. Primary Health Solutions want to provide high quality healthcare at a price and site that is convenient for all consumers, being payer agnostic with their services.

Frank Perez, former KHN CEO, reported on the Good Neighbor House, which is located downtown. It started 25 years ago, when six congregations started a Dorcas program. In the Adventist Church, the Biblical Dorcas provides a place where people can receive clothing. Frank was a recipient of these services in 1962 in a Maryland Dorcas Program, which helped him survive by receiving winter clothing. Peter was a pastor at one of those churches decades ago. All of the local six congregations were on the outskirts of Dayton but wanted to focus on the downtown area. They moved to their downtown site in 1994. They asked Wright State University to conduct a community assessment downtown, and dental services were a big need there, even for Medicaid patients. Even now, three million Ohioans lack dental care.

Good Neighbor House is a free clinic (sliding scale; patients come from all over the state) and provides dental care (anchor and teaching site; free consultation, referral center for crowns, root canals and advanced care), as well as medical care, special dietary support, clothing, and a thrift store. They have 450 participants in Wellness Classes. Special dietary staff enroll diabetic and hypertensive patients into a controlled environment with medical and nutrition services—they get a Kroger gift certificate card to receive foods appropriate for their specific health conditions.

Good Neighbor House is seeing lives change. A 44-year-old Hispanic man was bouncing from ED to ED within all hospitals. He crashed often, showing up with a 550 blood sugar level. At one ED, they sent him to the Good Neighbor House for sustained support. In July 2019, he came to their program with that high blood sugar level. They started insulin support and put him in the Wellness program. A few weeks ago, the volunteer medical provider saw him with a blood sugar of 119 and he's had no ED visits since July.

The Good Neighbor House receives no public funding, just runs from donations and philanthropy. It's God's work at its best. They re-located from their original site to a larger one recently.

Rev. Karen Young (Director of Dayton Scholars in West Dayton) had received a report about low functioning in terms of education, which spurred her to start the Dayton Scholars. Two hundred children come from various schools, working on increasing their social and emotional needs in terms of staying in school. They wish to restore the relationship between the teacher and child. Also, in Pre-K to 3rd grade, they need to improve math and reading literacy. They provide breakfast, lunch and snacks.

Their curriculum includes improving self-esteem and helping parents note that there is a problem earlier. Parents are low in literacy themselves and trying to survive more than thinking of caring for the children. They engage the parents in these efforts. The parents help with getting their Graduation Equivalency Diploma (GED), as well as reading to the children. There are 20-30 persons per site to help the children. The ratio of teacher-children is far too high in the schools. Dayton Scholars wants to improve the 15% 3rd grade reading level. Intense study helps. This is their 2nd year of operation.

Grandview blessed the Dayton Scholars in their efforts to bridge the gap in education. They need teachers who understand the stress of living in poverty. Grandview provided funding for special tutoring, map charts, ABC charts, food for the weekends and dinners, testing supplies, and some staff to help teach team building, sharing and respect. Dayton Scholars offer games like football and baseball, and science projects. The program costs $90K per year. Each child is afforded quiet time (just to read, do math, practice how to write legibly). Each child receives a full backpack and food.

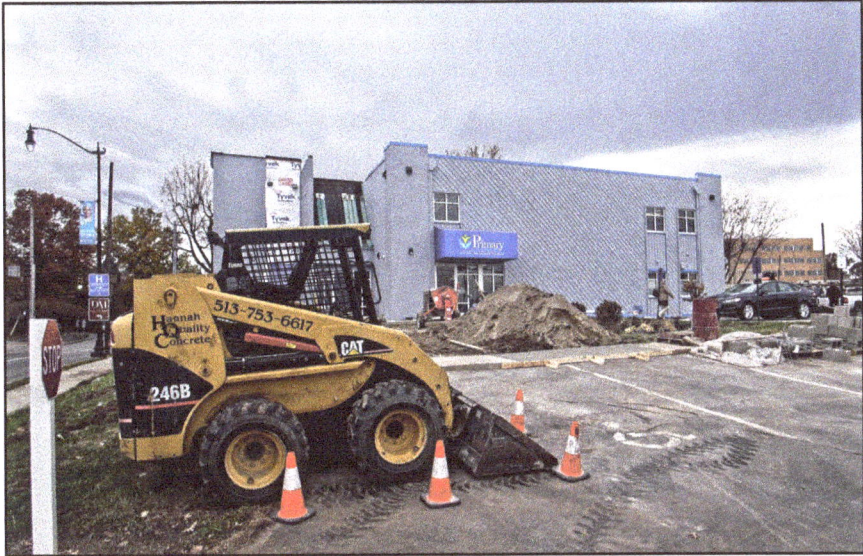

Dayton New Primary Health Solutions Clinic

Their wholistic approach helps their children have a good start, move away from crisis mode and have a great educational foundation. Dayton Scholars hosts four sites each year, taking 75 kids per site.

Tom Thompson shared about an African Church Ministry, a large community of immigrants who gather at a former Christian Scientist church, from the Democratic Republic of Congo, Rwanda, and other African countries. Most immigrants come here with three months' worth of support and then are left to their own devices. Tom shared that Bonnie Baker connected them to Wright State University, University of Dayton, Catholic Social Services, Public Health, Welcome Dayton and others providing resources to the immigrant society, to better map available resources. However, due to lingual or cultural competency barriers, when that 60-90 day support drops off, the individuals were still in need.

KHN has helped by, first, collaborating with a local non-profit that provides education in learning the English language by helping fund tutors, and second, getting jobs. Through the Oniru Group, Cross Over Community Development provides tutors for those who are illiterate in their own language (many lived their whole life in refugee camps, so their ability is limited). St. John's Church provides English as a Second Language (ESL) tutors to much of the refugee population who are literate in their own languages.

Several local organizations assist refugees in finding job opportunities and helping them bridge cultural barriers. Many immigrants have a hard time sustaining employment or even applying for jobs— it's difficult to describe a job history or understand work culture after living in a refugee camp all your life.

A small number of the refugee population have now gained employment at KHN, and KHN representatives work with Fidel, the pastor of the church, to trouble-shoot day to day issues. They are helping with legal aid, being an advocate, or a conduit to resources such as ESL or GED classes, healthcare, courts, police department, etc. INF helps, but you must register every six months.

Tom is starting a Foundation for 100 mentors to walk with immigrants, through friendship and understanding. Immigrants need a "go-to person" to avoid despair. Their philosophy is, "We won't leave you." Former CEO Becky Lewis went to the neighborhood and said, "KHN won't leave you," which carried much positive power.

Peter wants suburban churches to invest in urban ministries. He is working with the United Way to create a map around needed resources in local neighborhoods. Kathy Perno codified this model: clergy, congregation, larger community. At its center is Faith Community CARE Partners, who wish to improve the quality of life of all people in communities. They wish to convey God's love to all. Ministry Care Line is an EAP for clergy and their families to provide support.

In Middletown, the clergy said, "We are hurting. We are burnt out." They are helping clergy couples, too. Congregations will be provided access to CREATION Health and other educational offerings. The KHN team plans to track longitudinal data to show impact.

There are 5000 nurses in KHN. What if each one was offered a chance to work with their own congregations? This could grow quickly with a speaker's bureau and other offerings.

Indianapolis, Indiana

12. Near Northwest Faith Partners, Flanner House Community Center

https://iuhealth.org/

Contact: Rev. Dr. Jay Foster, Indiana University Health
38 Attendees, 16 male, 22 female; 18 White, 20 AA

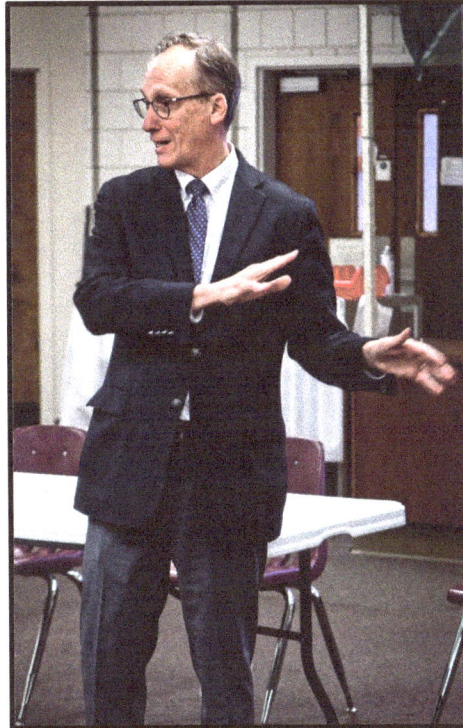

Jay Foster at Near Northwest
Faith Partners Meeting

This was a key Stakeholder meeting with Faith-Health partners, including IU Health Department of Spiritual Care, Congregational Partnerships, and congregational leaders. Paticipants were Congregational and Community Leaders Rev. Dr. Ivan Douglas Hicks, First Baptist Church, North Indianapolis; Andrew Green, Asst. Exec. Director, Shepherd Community Center; David Craig, PhD, Chair of Department of Religious Studies, IUPUI: Vern Farnum, Director AHC Chaplaincy, IU Health; Anastasia Holman, Manager, Chaplaincy Education, IU Health. The meeting included:

- Video presentation and Panel Discussion, Healthy Indiana Plan (HIP) Survey
- Presentation by Dr. Gary Gunderson on FaithHealth potential in Marion County

Rev. Ivan Douglas Hicks of First Baptist Church, North Indianapolis, facilitated the meeting, starting with a video of the Healthy Indiana Plan Members and Congregational Leaders. Study partners were the First Baptist Church North Indianapolis, the Shepherd Community Center, and IUPUI, and it was funded by the Indiana Minority Health Coalition. Ivan shared more about the Near Northwest Faith Partners coalition.

First Baptist Church has been a part of this neighborhood for 135 years now. The church, as the oldest social service agency in the neighborhood, is responsive to and responsible for their neighbors and their members. There have been increasing concerns about violence, lack of quality food, older homes, environmental problems, chronic diseases, and higher cancer rates in this area.

The church runs a soup kitchen and provides clothing and other services. Butler University, North Marion, IUPUI and other academic partners are close by. The neighborhood wanted to learn more about their own assets and issues. Holy Angel Catholic Church, Flanner House, and others work collaboratively to improve local residents' health.

Local residents shared their stories about the difficulty of accessing even basic health care and how those problems can exacerbate existing health problems. An advocate shared about the difficulties in accessing care for the homeless and why the ED often becomes the primary care home for them. Recommendations from those in the neighborhood were shared.

A panel discussion then also took place with Dr. David Craig, Chair of Religious Studies Dept., IUPUI, as well as Suzanne Coleman and Sheila Powell, members of First Baptist Church, North Indianapolis (stars of the video).

Suzanne shared that there is much work to do and they must keep hope alive. She had full health care coverage but moved to a part-time job and her coverage decreased in scope. God presented this HIP program opportunity, she believes. HIP wanted her to pay $10 to apply, which didn't guarantee coverage. She said she would be notified later, to see if received coverage or not. She received three letters, with the third one stating that she didn't qualify. Sheila is still not covered, but, thankfully, she has no health conditions at this time. However, she plans to try to apply again, during open enrollment.

Sheila shared more about her post-surgery experience. She had retired but had to return to work, which altered her healthcare premium costs from $20 to $107 per month. While she was upset at first, she realized that she still had full medical, vision and dental coverage, which makes her feel blessed. Suzanne said that "Obama made us go to the doctor," and she sees the value of regular maintenance and preventive care. Sheila does take a lot of medicine and, on HIP Plus, her co-pay was covered. Getting on the phone and finding the right representative (her phone has limited minutes) took forever. She had to negotiate a different form of insulin to avoid a co-pay of $25. It took two calls and an extra visit to the doctor to fix this, but it would have cut into her grocery budget if she had been required to meet that cost. Most older persons wouldn't be able to navigate this complexity.

Dr. David Craig shared his thanks that many had opened doors for him to do this study. In 2018, one in four persons who were on HIP lost coverage within a year. Many didn't understand why. HIP has to be applied for, used and reapplied for annually. Navigating the healthcare system is very complex.

In terms of wellness and what keeps you healthy, the factors named were food deserts, stigma, and mistrust. There is a historical mistrust of the healthcare institutions. You bridge that by being present, communicating, listening, and helping meet named needs. One person shared with David that a counselor, a nurse and others listened to his need, which was healing; this meant that HIP-Plus was value-added to him. This work requires partnership.

Rev. Dr. Jay Foster, VP of Spiritual Care & Congregational Partnerships for Indiana University Health, thanked all for coming and introduced Dr. Gary Gunderson. Gary shared more about Stakeholder Health, the Memphis Model, and the trust issue in improving health. Gary then asked what issues were top priority for those in the room.

Rev. Hicks stated that Indianapolis has lead levels exceeding many other deeply affected areas, especially if your home was built before 1974 when regulations came into place. They need to educate and make residents aware of lead poisoning symptoms and differentiate these from symptoms of ADHD or other problems, some of which appear similar. Testing needs to be done. Faith communities can move into this area of work. There are parents who fear having their children tested, for fear that the authorities will take their children or, if they find high lead levels, they will be subjected to fines and more.

Rev. Hicks and others have been talking with IUPUI about conducting the testing for lead in dust, soil, and water. Those results come back to the homeowner first. Gary Holland, the NAACP representative, and others have done work in New Jersey about lead poisoning prevention legislation and the group here will meet with them later tonight.

Franciscan Health is looking at Adverse Childhood Experiences (ACES), building communities of resilience, and trauma-informed care, which should be helpful in improving community health.

Jay Foster shared that he wants to listen, learn from what has already been done by Rev. Hicks, David Craig, and many others in Marion County. This effort to deeply listen will inform the pilot program that Jay wants to conduct. As in Memphis and Wake Forest, you start by listening and building a covenant of sorts. Jay and IUH will work with ten congregations to accompany people and help them navigate the complex healthcare system.

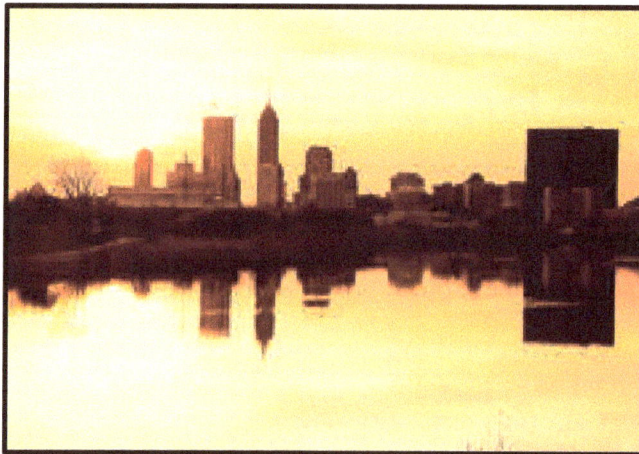

Friday, Nov. 22, 2019

Indianapolis, Indiana

13. Grassroots Maternal and Child Health Leadership
     Training Project: Riley Children's Foundation Infant
     Mortality Prevention Program

https://www.rileykids.org/

Contacts: Dr. Nancy Swigonski and Dr. Jack Turman

4 Attendees, 3 male, 1 female; All White

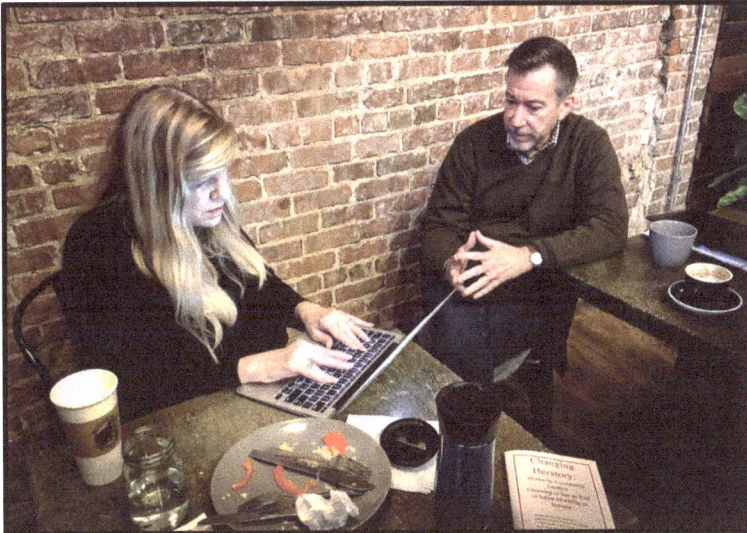

Teresa Cutts and Jack Turman

Dr. Nancy Swigonski and Dr. Jack Turman shared about the Riley Children's Foundation's sponsored infant mortality prevention program, the Grassroots Maternal and Child Health Leadership Training Project. This program trains and mentors women to help their neighborhoods improve pregnancy and infant development outcomes. They work to make change at the community, organizational and policy levels, while meeting the needs of women, infants, and families in their neighborhoods by linking them to services. Jay Foster and Csaba Szilagyi, Chaplain Manager at Riley Children's Hospital, also attended.

Gary shared briefly about Winston Salem's fledgling age 0-3 initiative and solicited their advice. Nancy is a senior pediatrician and health services researcher. An initial statewide project was addressing the long wait list for children needing autism (or on the spectrum) assessment and diagnosis. At that time, the average age of diagnosis was 5.6 years old. They set up a hub of centers and were funded by the Riley Children's Foundation to train primary care providers to make these diagnoses.

To date, they've now seen over 2,000 children across the state. Nancy's efforts now all focus on infant mortality, but there is an intersection with early childhood development and a recognition that it is a key stage in future health status. For infant mortality, if one looks at an analysis of Perinatal Periods of Risk (PPOR), one can view the causes from an epidemiological standpoint.

The analysis divides babies into those that are born under 1500 grams (~3 pounds) and by the time of death (fetal, neonatal, or infant). Being born weighing less than 1500 grams is associated with poorer outcomes. The PPOR analysis then compares a standard reference group of White women with more than HS education and private insurance, who have very low infant mortality rates, to everyone else —the difference is called the "excess mortality". If you wish to make a real impact, you must address the causes of "excess mortality", which are Maternal health (not maternal obstetrical care) and infant health (not NICU care). To have healthy babies, you must have healthy moms; to have healthy moms, you must have healthy communities. We must build networks in high risk communities where "people are willing to trust (not just be educated), learn and change behavior."

Jack shared that Nancy has done a great job of taking a community-based approach to deal with healthy infants/moms to complement excellent, traditional medical care. Building capacity of childcare centers was a key. They went into one of the highest areas of disparity and high infant mortality (there are big local geographic differences in Indiana and Indianapolis). The community said they wanted childcare options. This was daunting, but it makes perfect sense.

Nancy's group obtained a Kohl's community-based grant to look at barriers to high quality and accessible childcare. One factor was that providers didn't have the right materials or supplies for a high-quality licensed childcare for early infant care (such as a rocking chair, fridge, and other materials). Lots of excellent work was going on in the community but it focused primarily on pre-schoolers and not infants. They collaborated with multiple community and state partners such as United Way, the Office of Early Childhood, and Early Learning Indiana.

Despite the great work that was happening, when partners came together no one was closing the loop on whether they actually connected; no tracking occurred. Their initiative started tracking these connections. There were already quality rating coaches who could do the audits to direct what was needed in the centers. They found that centers often under-reported their needs, and that developmentally appropriate and safe sleep materials were the highest needs. They started with an average need of $4500 per center; then the centers could build their quality rating, which then allowed more positive cycles of centers improving quality and building capacity. To date, they have worked with 82 early child and infant care centers.

They found phenomenal individuals in the community. One childcare provider was doing financial counseling for her families and she had limited education herself. Now she is a superstar in the program and works for the initiative eight hours per week, building a network of childcare providers. She started her center at level 1 (lowest level), then went up to quality level 3 (high quality), and is working to go to level 4 (national accreditation).

Gary asked how many centers or initiatives are run by faith communities? Some of the larger ones, we were told, are run by faith leaders but, generally, they are "exempt" and may not meet quality standards because of the physical structure of the buildings.

The initiative is now expanding up to Fort Wayne and their business leaders are anxious to get moving, but understand that the effort has to be driven by the community and with community partners, so they are patient on local start up.

Jack started his career as a developmental neuroscientist, studying fetal and infant brain development. Several influential neuroscientists crafted ideas about moving to community level—"neurons to neighborhoods and others"—and now Jack is a community activist in terms of maternal and child health, going from the lab to the "hood". Only here for just over two years, he met Nancy and they bonded in terms of wanting to take action at the community level to improve infant mortality rates. His emphasis is to shift the focus and narrative of infant mortality from the individual level to the societal level. His work is place-based and goes to where infant mortality rates are historically high. It is time, he said, to focus on changing social, political, economic, and environmental factors that consistently contribute to poor birth outcomes.

Jack and his team work to train and mentor community women to be grassroots maternal and child health leaders. They recruit women from socially high-risk neighborhoods, from re-entry programs, from affordable housing communities, or from other agencies providing care for marginalized women. The women identified are trusted, compassionate women in a neighborhood, but are not in everyone's business.

He doesn't recruit grasstops leaders (those on every Board, in everyone's business). His cohort of workers have to be out there and embedded in the neighborhoods. TC asked, "How do you deal with political pushback on not recruiting the grasstops leaders?" Jack says that this is a big problem, but lots of different people are needed to do this work. His answer is "We work alongside you to complement your efforts."

Now, 18 months later, Jack's program has 14 women from eight different zip codes working. Ten of the women make less than $10K per year. This cohort has been trained through a curriculum aimed to create social change leaders, not community health workers. The curriculum was recently published in the ENGAGE! journal. Each grassroots maternal and child health leader learns: professional storytelling (oral and written) to influence community members and policy and decision makers; to survey communities and then bridge evidence based programs into their own communities; to give high impact TED Talk presentations to thought leaders; and, to develop and advocate for policies. His cohort don't want to have only incremental impact, but sustainable social change that benefits all women, babies and families.

A media team produces YouTube and professional videos to spread the word about this initiative (see, for example: https://youtu.be/vHLZMzFLxv8, https://youtu.be/5a5-rymyTRY, http://www.youtube.com/watch?v=owcSnuXIH5A).

.

14. Shepherd Community Center

https://www.shepherdcommunity.org/

Contact: Andrew Green, Assistant Executive Director
5 Attendees, 4 male, 1 female; 4 White, 1 AA

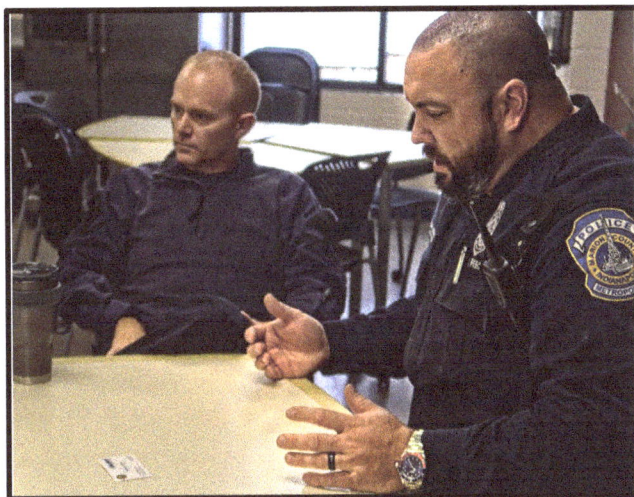

Shane Hardwick and Adam Perkins

The Shepherd Community Center (SCC), is a 34 year initiative of the Church of the Nazarene on the Near North East side, but now features a new ministry in which they employ an Indianapolis Police Department officer and an emergency medicine technician (Paramedic) to go round in the neighborhood.

After welcoming us, Mr. Green led a tour of SCC, and this was followed by a discussion with police officers, Emergency Medial Technicians (EMT), and leaders of faith and health initiatives embedded in the community that Shepherd serves. In addition to serving as Assistant Executive Director, Mr. Green is a lay leader in the church. Shepherd Center goes to the community instead of community members always coming to the Center. The neighborhood had been mapped for incidence of violence by Indianapolis Metro Police Dept., with a hotspot one mile from SCC. The police department approached SCC to ask them to work with a paramedic and law enforcement person in zip codes 46201 and 46203, where about 165,000 persons reside. The police department's primary objective is to concentrate their efforts within a 1-2 mile radius. Adam Perkins (Police Dept. reserve) and Shane Hardwick (paramedic) shared about their work, responding initially to community calls, but, more importantly, doing follow up visits.

This is a unique partnership; SCC hired these two persons. Four and a half years ago, Adam Perkins was ignoring God's call on his life and was unhappy in the corporate world. He answered a second e-mail, soliciting his current work. He didn't know what to do, so they told him "Be Norm from Cheers." He had been a reserve officer, mostly shaking hands, kissing babies, and taking 9-1-1 calls.

This neighborhood has all the negative demographics of many underserved communities: lots of single moms and elderly. It was the 3rd most violent neighborhood in Indianapolis when they started, with lots of predatory businesses and intergenerational poverty. Adam found that, if he was able to spend time listening and building relationships, he began to make headway on some of those problems. Adam shared more. The second shift for the police department in this neighborhood is the busiest beat in the country (per capita), and most guys working it are new on the force and aim to go somewhere else as fast as they can. The average citizen calling 9-1-1 gets an average of 4.5 minutes with a police officer. Like the complaints about seeing a physician, that's not enough time.

Adam began to change that visit time statistic. For him, the average on scene time at the beginning was 28.4 minutes, which helped a lot. That was the initial visit. In that 28 minutes, he gives his business card with a cell number. He often met a lonely, desperate person who can call him if in need in the future. The mental health and substance use disorder (SUD) or health related stuff was still problematic. About 6 months into Adam's work, Eskanzi Health and Hospitals' umbrella hired Shane to help. Their first agreement was that they would not overpromise and under-deliver in the community. Often there is grant work, then the community is left when the money runs out.

The poverty problem is huge. Intergenerational poverty teaches people to get food stamps and disability income. Beyond that, they have limited skills. Adam and Shane began to help persons access new resources. SCC allows the duo to engage their calling in a way that is so important. SCC is unique in that they often say "yes" when they don't know how to do something and are not afraid to fail. SCC's network is very deep, and they are respected here. SCC also don't have to own everything, and their mantra is "community impact through collaboration." There have been times when there is a community tragedy, and Adam moves into the space of a chaplain. His wife had a wooden sign made for him, with his quote: "Law enforcement done right looks more like ministry than law."

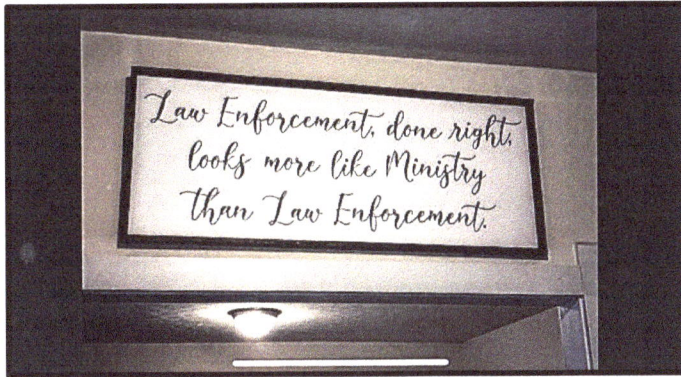

Adam Perkins' Law Enforcement and Ministry Quote

Shane did emergency medical services (EMS) for inner city 25 years and loved it, mostly working on gunshot wounds, accidents: "Running and gunning." Having a front row seat to see what poverty does and seeing how people raise their kids, he became "beyond jaded." He questioned his faith and humanity, developed a negative perspective and swore he'd never come back here. From an EMS perspective, if you keep picking up the same folks over and over again, you wonder "Why are you going back to the hospital repeatedly?"

Shane worked as an administrator for a few years, and this opportunity to work with Adam arose and they posed this question to patients, "Why do you keep going back to the hospital?" He realized that, after becoming embedded in the neighborhood, there is good stuff going on as well as the bad. Adam and Shane's team identify people in need in the initial 9-1-1 call and people are a bit put off by the big police department officer. For example, the call is for pneumonia, so the patient asks, "Why is there a policeman here? "After the ambulance comes, the team looks deeper to the root causes of why the same persons keep calling. High ED utilizers are asked "Why do you keep coming back to the hospital?" The team now thinks that the root causes are one of many social determinants of health issues: social work issue, Medicaid issue, transportation, behavioral health issue, SUD issue, patient-care related.

The healthcare system only works if a person can make it to a doctors' office or other healthcare setting. Transportation is an issue. IUH has a case management person in this neighborhood, while

Eskanzi has a patient care navigator and social worker at another hospital. A lot of Adam and Shane's work is knocking on folks' doors and then following up. "Did you get your medications, your follow up appointments, etc.?" Persons often don't understand discharge instructions and the team helps with that issue. They have a van component to transport persons to appointments. Their theme for this year is trying to eliminate the transactional and replace it with the relational. There are so many roadblocks put in the way by the transactional nature of how healthcare is delivered. For example, a lady who needed Medicaid rides had to fill out a long form that a phone operator had to complete. She was in her 40's, had her first heart attack at 36, was not able to breathe, bent over from pain, had only fans in window and it was over 100 degrees in her unit. She kept ending up in the ICU every few days. A donor gave an air conditioner (AC) unit after seeing their newspaper article. The team perceived getting an AC for this lady as a God thing. As this woman got her AC installed, air was blowing on her and she was bawling with gratitude.

Their team began to see the patterns of human behavior. One man was in a unit with no doorknob and had abdominal pain a few weeks prior. The man has gastrointestinal esophageal reflux disease and needs Zantac. When it runs out for him, the 3rd week of the month, he was using the ED for primary care to his drugs refilled. Adam and Shane got his meds for him, a pill box, a regular primary care doctor and he still may need an assessment for developmental delays. Hopefully, their team can get him to his primary care provider and he'll get what he needs, and they'll hand his care off to others.

There is an issue of replicating the program. Community paramedicine is a one-trick pony—call them and haul them. In terms of law enforcement, jail and prison are not the answer. They are trying to educate the community. Officer Perkins is just as concerned about congestive heart failure as Shane is concerned about drug sales and prostitution. It's all public health.

They met a guy yesterday who was gruff and cursing. He said, "I wish people would leave me alone." He pays for everything and hides in the back bedroom, while his kids and grandkids bring their lower quality of life friends to his house. None have a job. This is his existence. He is extremely lonely. The Anthem Health guy rode along to see this. If the man could feel better, he might not be passively suicidal. They have had a few chaplain and clergy ride along. As Shane deals with the health component, Adam is in the background, looking at the social and other factors. Yesterday, went for a welfare check and the lady was feeling suicidal. She had assaulted her husband a few days before. She had her meds changed and her nephew had jumped off a bridge a few weeks before. She needs grief counseling and more. Now her medications are being adjusted and they are providing support.

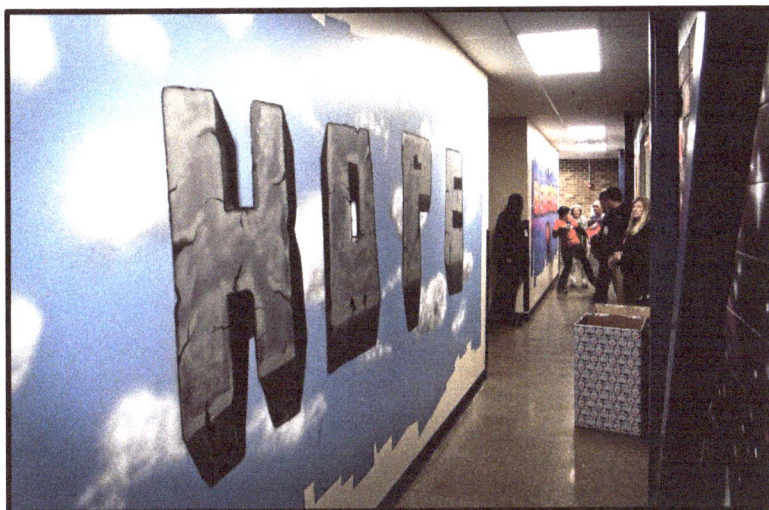

Hope Mural at Shepherd Center, Indianapolis

Those two examples above exemplify an integrated approach. They debrief and have a bigger wholistic picture. Another police officer had given more context and background on the woman's case. They see that they may need to do more. There is a faith-based Celebrate Recovery program here and Adam is the minister for it. They have tried to replicate the Quick Response Team (QRT), found in Huntington and work with the hospital. They've had many dealings with folks who are addicted and develop relationships with them, often using McDonald gift cards as currency to get them a hot lunch. SCC has a family ministry team and they meet with them in terms of increasing accountability—a full community-based team approach.

Unless they have promised a follow up on a given day, Adam and Shane don't have a set schedule and just naturally make their rounds. They are expanding their circles to include other case managers. They do make birthday calls, which helps people who are so lonely. A 94-year-old lady has a lung condition and anxiety and she really just wants them to just "Stay awhile." They went by to check on her and noticed that two calls were flagged: Christmas and New Year's Eve. So their team worked on bringing others in to provide visits for her.

Shane shared a visual of the blue bar ED visits pre-involvement and red bar ED visits post-involvement, with a significant decrease in visits. Their team are not babysitters or handlers and don't enable those they serve. The folks they serve live in a house of cards, with incredibly complex lives. They educate and empower. They recently saw a couple, married for 40 years. The husband has dementia and they want to stay in the house. The couple's ramp has a bump in it, so they called Servants of Ministry, who build wheelchair ramps. Adam and Shane discovered that the ministry didn't want to fix the ramp, because the couple really needed to go to assisted living. The lady was then motivated to fix up the house to sell it for a profit. If you don't have a ground game, you don't understand the depth of the needs OR how the usual "fixes" enable things negatively.

They have a holiday donor who helps annually. They thought about using those funds to help a family who knows how to work the system to get what they need. Unfortunately, the family hasn't stepped up to do anything to help themselves. The man in the family has a SUD, alcohol. The team went to the local liquor store owner and asked them to bar the guy from the liquor store. At 8:30 the next morning, the man is there. The team had warned him the day before that they were going to shut down his access to alcohol and went to the other local stores to stop his behavior. The man was going to ED for hydration after a hangover and hit an officer on probation. After that, for six months he did well and was sober. Then the man started drinking again, they took him in to his probation officer and shared that he was drinking. They offer tough and inconvenient and assertive love.

They spend much time with folks they visit. They trained the mobile unit crisis assessment team (MCAT). Adam and Shane were not allowed to do formal crisis calls, couldn't do the follow up MCAT visits. They see the follow up, relationship with SCC and time spent with people as differentiators from MCAT work. Best results come when Adam and Shane make that first visit. There are some folks who are too volatile to do that first call with the MCAT. They just log that person mentally and expect they will see them again for other issues.

Shane went to a presentation and the group was fixated on transportation, thinking only about what the most reliable form of transport was. Shane noted that churches are key there, tying that need into that desire to serve. However, there is often a disconnect between church volunteers and where they will go. Perhaps the team could leverage their trust by proxy, and they could vet and match volunteers with those they serve.

15. Community Clinic at Redeemer Church, Monroe County FaithHealth Efforts

https://redeemerbloomington.org/

Contact: Jay Foster
Tour of Redeemer Church Clinic, followed by discussion
with local stakeholders

6 Attendees, 4 male, 2 female; All White

Emily Manlove, Jesse Taylor, Shawn Gerber, Tim Jensen, Jay Foster

Congregational and Community Leaders: Carol Weiss-Kennedy, Director, Community Health, IU Health Bloomington; Shawn Gerber, Director, Spiritual Care, IU Health, Bloomington; Emily Manlove, MD, hospitalist, IU Health Bloomington and IU Health Southern Indiana Physicians; Rev. Jesse Taylor of Redeemer Church

Bloomington, IN, has a population of 110,000 in Monroe County, with 40,000 of those being students at IUH-Bloomington. IU Health is the major provider in the area. They provide maternal and child health for eleven counties, with the rural counties having poorer infant mortality and teen pregnancy rates. Monroe County is the only Democratic county in Indiana.

IUH-Bloomington's Community Health Division is led by Health Educator, Director Carol Weiss-Kennedy. The department began in 1996 with registered nurses, nurse practitioners, registered dieticians, health educators, and more. They run the HIV/AIDs clinical programs with funding sources through the Indiana State Department of Health, Ryan White funds, and the Health Foundation of Greater Indianapolis. This includes prevention, care coordination, housing, treatment, and substance use disorder (SUD) treatment. They serve Monroe County and 49 of 92 Indiana counties (an initiative called Positive Link).

They also have HUD money for transitional supportive housing and long-term and permanent housing. Nurse Family Partnerships provides home visits to eligible mothers and infants, is the sponsoring agent for WIC, and has 82 staff. It runs Alzheimer's Resource Services and provides clinical services for the Monroe County Health Department. The Community Health Department also provides tobacco prevention, diabetes, and medical nutrition therapy (it can bill for diabetes education and medical nutrition therapy). Total budget is $5.5M; $700K comes from the hospital. Their offices are not on hospital grounds. IUH-Bloomington is building a new hospital facility on the eastern side of the city, which will be a regional academic health center.

In Bloomington, Centerstone, a not-for-profit housed in Nashville, provides behavioral health and is trying to become a FQHC look-alike. Volunteers in Medicine will become a FQHC and provide primary care and dentistry services. In Monroe County, IUB provides EMS. Wheeler Mission, the homeless shelter, is down the street with a fire department located nearby. The EMS Director wants to look at high utilizers, like one lady who has called 75 times to go to the ED in the last few months, so they are planning proactive visits. Monroe County is a very collaborative community with no ownership issues. Monroe Hospital is a small (24 bed), for-profit facility, offering the only other inpatient facility in the County.

Rev. Shawn Gerber is the Director of Spiritual Care and Chaplaincy Services at IU Health Bloomington Hospital. He is the Chaplain Manager for the IU Health South Central region, which includes IU Health Morgan Hospital in Morgan County, IU Health Bedford Hospital in Lawrence County, and IU Health Paoli Hospital in Orange County, working across Monroe, Morgan, Orange (Mennonite and Amish population), and Lawrence rural counties. Shawn is ordained in the Mennonite Church USA and attends the Mennonite Fellowship of Bloomington and First United Methodist Church in Bloomington. There is one Mennonite Church USA congregation in Paoli (Orange County), in addition to conservative Mennonite and Amish communities spread across the rural areas of Orange County. IU-B has eight catchment counties and is a Level 3 Trauma Center. There is partisan divide in terms of where people go for hospital service.

Rev. Jesse Taylor is a pastor at Redeemer Community Church (RCC). He helped with the initial development of the Care Clinic and Mercy Team. Bloomington is a place that offers a lot of services, especially for a small city, probably related to it housing a major university. As a result, many homeless and folks living in intergenerational poverty come here for those services. RCC wanted to bridge the gap between local congregations and mercy ministry. There are parachurch ministries, but RCC wanted to really get involved in the community, getting their ideas from Michigan City Christ Church and learning from them.

RCC started their first Care Clinic in 2016. They have a unique advocate role—a person who walks folks through all the services and ends by offering a shared meal. Its overall mission is to have persons involved at the church, but they serve anyone. Their Fall 2016 Care Clinic started with non-emergency medical assistance (RN, MD and others). Redeemer Community Church holds these clinics three times a year. IUB brought their Health Mobile to offer more services. Until then, they had hosted about 200 persons in their Back to School clinic. November clinics usually host about 100 persons; this year 300 people came. Sixty people were lined up before they opened. Vendors come to offer services, and one can find Medicaid enrollment, social services, hygiene and personal supplies, diapers, toilet paper, and haircuts (especially for kids).

RCC wants to see what is needed and bridge that need, with an emphasis on respect and dignity. When they do their volunteer training (N=53), they say the goal is NOT efficiency, but to slow down and get to know folks. Over time, they saw the need for follow up medical care. They also started a food pantry, offer cups of coffee, hygiene supplies, and other resources (community care management). "Jesus truly loves this work," they say; members of RCC are driven by their faith. Of course, many churches started hospitals and clinics, but there has been a disconnect over the years. RCC wants to care for the whole person, and has 4 paid FTEs, 2 part-time staff, and an intern. They have about 450 regular attendees on Sunday. April, August, and November are generally when they hold their Care Clinics. The need is great and they have repeat persons who come, especially for back to school offerings. They get a handful of persons from surrounding counties too, and as people who live in poverty learn about services, they start coming. What RCC does is fairly easily replicated at other churches.

RCC moved to the current site about 18 months ago. Bloomington Baptist Church sold them the building and most of their 20 members (average age was 70) came to be part of their congregation. They are affiliated with a couple of church planting networks but are Reformed Baptists (similar to Presbyterians in terms of polity, but adhering to Believer's baptism). Hotels donate shampoo and other supplies. Mother Hubbard's Cupboard donates diapers, and Community Health hosts a Diaper Dash annually in which people enroll by bringing diapers. In the first year of the Diaper Dash, diapers were required to register, but going forward the team found that they could purchase diapers through the hospital at a lower cost. So now they ask for a $20 registration fee, which goes to purchase the diapers as well as other items that new families might need. Connections help with resources for the Care Clinics and makes the work more sustainable. RCC's move to this site helped them be in a more central epicenter for community-based care.

The question was posed: "Is there anything going on in Bloomington that requires that deep level of work in the community?" At RCC, they partner with Wheeler Mission to help folks struggling with addictions and homelessness get plugged into a church community. There is a crisis response team locally, run by Centerstone in partnership with law enforcement, but faith communities haven't been part of this. There is a new crisis diversion unit for behavioral health and SUD, opening in early 2020. This is a great example of community collaboration between IU Health, Centerstone, Monroe County Government, and others. Cook Medical is the biggest employer in Monroe County, making a variety of medical devices, but couldn't get a decent workforce to stay on site. Now Cook offers help for employees to obtain their GED and other services. So, the current BH/SUD crisis service offerings that are opening also were driven by the workforce need.

There is a convergence of energy in the state around faith and health work. At a recent meeting of the Bloomington Area Interfaith Alliance, a need for medical transportation was named (200 folks need rides to dialysis, etc.). The Bloomington Health Foundation wonders how faith communities could help stand in the gap. Leslie Levine, President of the Congregation Beth Shalom, has been involved in these discussions. As a community, traditionally, the faith comunities don't work well together. This may have to do with conservative and liberal divisions among faith traditions. TC shared that in Huntington, West VA, these theological differences were transcended as clergy worked together to address the opioid crisis.

Emily Manlove, a family physician/hospitalist for IUH-B, moved here with her husband a few years ago and was drawn to RCC before they had a building. The Nov. 2019 Care Clinic was her first as a volunteer where she saw 18 patients and wrote four prescriptions for asthma and a few other conditions. Five needed follow up and had been seen at IUH-B; two were transient and had moved here recently but couldn't access primary care until many months out. There is a primary care provider shortage, so Emily will try to get those persons' medication refilled before that initial visit. The Care Clinic is episodic, but providers can triage and advocate for patients. It is a casual environment, so patients may share more than average with a provider. Monroe County has Riley Physicians for pediatrics, who have better access to care than adults in the primary care realm.

Rev. Tim Jessen is an ordained Presbyterian minister who teaches and writes for the Religion Section, Herald Times, a one pager that comes out on Saturday. He is also affiliated with the Mennonite Fellowship of Bloomington and notes (through reviewing the Herald Times obituaries) how many persons die without a faith connection and/or service. The old church structures are dying; perhaps the new church is emerging, he said. People are hungry to engage faith and deed together. Healthcare itself is in crisis and needs to "remember who they are." Providers went into health to care for others, but, if health care can be delivered without efficiency, them it will probably be more healing for humans.

What does the Care Clinic need? Jesse says they need resources and staffing to offer more Care Clinics. Efficiency is not a part of the work; it's about relationship building. However, help bridging the need for medications or other care while awaiting an initial primary care visit would be good. Longer hours (against their current 10-12) might work better. Haircuts may also be a draw. Carol's staff, who were testing for HIV/AIDS at the most recent Care Clinic, said there wasn't much stigma. Her staff could arrange to block a few new clinic slots for those who need care, to provide continuity of care.

The Care Clinic follow up survey results identify what persons say they need and RCC tries to address these needs. Many people show up at the Food Pantry which James, their full-time intern, runs and he is an advocate to direct people to resources. RCC provides help with bills and utilities on a small scale. From RCC's perspective, living out the Good News in both word and deed is powerful. This attracts a certain type of membership.

Open Door Ministry, a worship service connected with First United Methodist of Bloomington, meets at the Buskirk Chumley Theater downtown. They also reach out to all in community, to "come as you are" (arm of United Methodist Church) and hold a revival in early December. Stinesville is a small town on the outskirts of Monroe County—very rural, very poor, and many residents deal with SUD. It is so small that it only has a Nazarene Church and general store. A few years ago, a parish nurse, Amy (who also manages Carol's Nurse Family Partnership), started a soccer team there and it is very popular on Tuesdays and Thursdays. They also offer foster care. The elementary school was closed and is empty. Amy wants to get women off the streets, out of domestic violence relationships and human trafficking. So they leased 30 beds in the school to start her new 501c3. Her ministry efforts were kick-started by police officers who called to get a woman out of human trafficking.

One woman with endocarditis has been in the hospital after long term SUD, and Shawn asked if she had a church connection. She had been to Care Clinic before, so Shawn will make the connection with Pastor Taylor. RCC has a good relationship with Wheeler Mission, which offers intensive SUD treatment and other structure, such as help with housing, etc. It can be difficult for persons to make that transition to other settings. RCC offers a way for people to enter easily into church life here.

Jay notes that Spiritual Care, traditionally, has been bedside only. He wants to expand chaplaincy to offer a spiritual care discharge plan. Via grant-funding, he is working to decrease social isolation. Shawn was "voluntold" by Jay (his boss) to host those interfaith pastors at the Community Outreach offices. Working together provides that common denominator that helps pastors learn about one another and care for the same folks out in community. In the new models of chaplaincy, they found that the chaplains also cared for the First Responders. Offering services for others makes those who serve healthier and happier and less jaded.

ENDINGS AND BEGINNINGS

Traveling for nearly three weeks we covered a lot of pavement, but also saw and paid attention to patterns we had never fully noticed before

From the very first thought of the very first See2See Road Trip, we were aiming for a fundamentally different way of learning than is available at even the most professional of national meetings. The problem is obvious: a profession comes with an official set of lenses and approved vocabulary for what is actually a ragged, chaotic and emergent phenomenon called "community." Which professional lens and language is appropriate? If you go to these kinds of meetings, you'll quickly notice that all of them are trying to think and talk in a new way about the same thing— the reality on the other side of the sidewalk from the hospital, public health office, community financial office, or Mayor's office (not to mention the hot mess in Washington!).

Imagine four big conference centers lined up in some metropolis surrounded by nice hotels for all the conventioneers. Those attending the APHA, AHA, IHI, NCL, NAS, NEA, or JPM will be hard to tell apart as they approach their respective meetings. But once inside they become almost unintelligible to each other as they rattle their acronyms and flash their PowerPoints until they wear out and head back to their hotels in the evening.

What they are all trying to talk about in their own arcane ways lies beyond the hotels where the neighborhoods sprawl with entire square miles of mystery. Mystery A: why are our professional meetings so extraordinarily expensive with such unimpressive results? A Norwegian friend, visiting one of our most esteemed hospitals, noted how remarkable it is that we accomplish so little with so much. Mystery B: Why, despite so many bands of professionals, do we continue as a society to slide further from justice with so many of our citizens nearly out of reach even of mercy?

Both mysteries lie in between the professional way of meeting, learning and talking. For the first coast-to-coast See2See that got us in a Winnebago in the first place, as we headed north and away from the APHA meeting in San Diego, then east—without PowerPoints, dim conference rooms, or even microphones. This time, we went a click more radical and left the Winnebago, too, replaced by a Mini Cooper getting 45 miles to the gallon. And in order to avoid the jet fuel, we planned a 1,700-mile loop, up and around the land the First People called the Inland Sea. For millennia, these mountains, huge rivers and vast lakes and endless hardwood forests were the cradle of the First civilized life on the continent. Archeologists tell us that the confluence of the Ohio, Kanawha, and Guyandotte rivers now called Huntington after a railroad baron, has been a trading settlement for at least 10,000 years. Epidemiologists know this and other river towns up and downstream are the epicenter of the deaths of despair.

This, perhaps, raises Mystery C: how did so much industrial wealth leave so little behind for the next generation to work with? Why did it take away even our hope, work, and self-respect as a people?

We could imagine a well-spent career exploring those mysteries along these roads over the mountains and through the woods of the Inland Sea. We only spent seven days, which is only a lot compared to the average professional meeting noted above. And we rode past some painfully interesting other towns with much to teach (Pittsburgh, Akron, Columbus, Louisville, Cincinnati were all *almost* on the route). What we saw even in this brief set of visits was all about extraordinary emergence where you'd least expect it, hope where the literature anticipated despair.

Like any travelers, we see through lenses we brought from home. Stakeholder Health people mostly live on the other side of the sidewalk all the time, even if our paychecks have a hospital logo. And we are tuned to the Leading Causes of Life, a language and logic born on the tough streets of Memphis and in southern Africa. Huntington, which some find scary, reminded us fondly of home. We thought of Aaron Antonovsky, the Jewish sociologist working after World War Two with women who had survived the death camps, raising children amid the bitter wars of the early Israeli state. He assumed struggle and trauma as the human norm; the mystery for him was health. How was *that* ever possible amid the baseline of human suffering and the horrors we do to each other over and over again? His answer created the field of *salutogenesis*, the seed of Leading Causes of Life. He would have recognized what we heard in Huntington, Cleveland, Dayton and Bloomington. For him, the most important quality a person, family, or community needs is not money for professional interventions to fix all that troubles one, but *coherence*.

Where the grown-ups in a place have a story that makes sense of the trauma—without fixing it—life has a chance. Nobody in these cities talked about the glory days of rail, steel, or auto, even though the streets are full of glorious left-behind architecture and vast tracts of abandoned factories. In Huntington, almost every story begins or rests on the 1970 crash of the Marshall team plane with 75 young men and many city leaders. The sorrow remains palpable.

But so is the almost animal tenacity that bonds people here together and makes it impossible for them to quit on each other, the city, or any of its most tragic and despairing members. It is not surprising to find Huntington a victim of one more cynical scheme such as opioids. And, once you know of the deep bonds that cohere in this place, you aren't surprised by the astonishing, creative, effective responses that have emerged here, either. Things happen here that are simply impossible to imagine in places with less coherence.

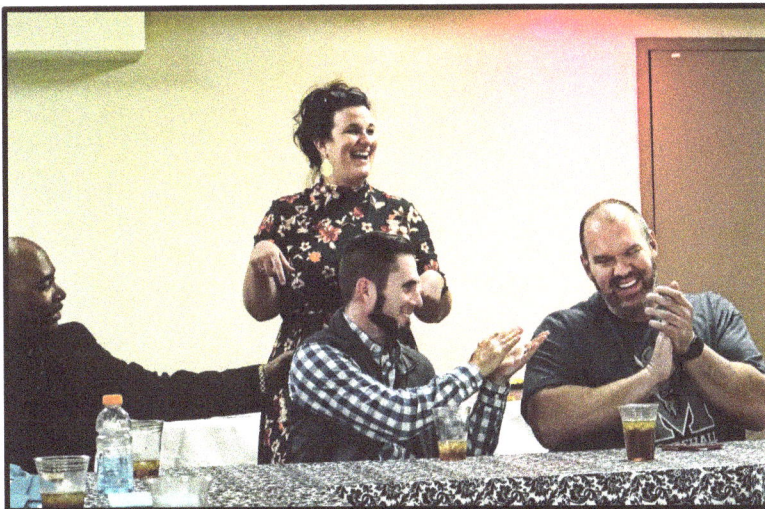

Some of the Quick Response Team, Huntington

The Quick Response Team is iconic in its simplicity: four people go and knock on every door of every person who has survived an overdose. They give a peanut butter sandwich, some brochures, and condoms. But also way more: the team includes a trained volunteer pastor who offers prayer, when it seems like it might be welcome (often is). And the team offers a pathway to real treatment real fast, like that night. The promise of fast real treatment rests on the extraordinary coherence of all relevant agencies and networks.

Even in the context of the utter and total evaporation of West Virginia's coal-based economy, the human networks are able to connect the frayed threads of the safety net to make that nighttime offer of treatment real. West Virginia has *less* of almost everything you would want in place. Instead it has way more of what turns out to be the essence of health—as Antonovsky would predict. The community is coherent. It is there for its members, even, maybe especially, those with the very least hope of all.

This is what we saw in various levels of radicality in each of the visits. Things work when people lean *out* of their professional identities *into* the humanity of their communities. They see beyond the list of interventions they could do to the obviously distressed neighborhoods, and see with a wider spectrum of possibilities.

In Cleveland, a city fallen much farther from its heights with all the same Huntington woes, the hospitals are among the very best in the world. That's not that most remarkable thing. One of them, University Health, followed its most vulnerable mothers and kids out of the doors of its excellent Rainbow Children's Hospital back to the deeply troubled neighborhoods and built a truly amazing center right there. Not entirely unlike Huntington, people are connected there in ways that go way beyond the negotiated plans. They are there for each other and won't quit.

Our favorite conversation for all 1,700 miles was with the security guy at the new Rainbow Center, who proudly pointed out his aunt's apartment across the street and recommended the new grocery story on the other corner. You could feel the pride of a man who worked for a place that was relevant to the neighbors, that had a coherent story for what was happening.

That is exactly the same pride we felt in the leadership of Evergreen, the largest organic hydroponic farm we've ever seen. The story, again, is about building a new company on the strong relationships of trust, not just cleverness. Everything the cooperative company does rests on and nurtures the sense of coherence that makes innovation and business growth possible. Any business has to get the books, machines and marketing right.

This business is built toward the very long arc—the one Martin King called justice—so it is careful about how all the employee-owners are related to the stakeholders (hospitals and local philanthropy) and customers (including Nestle) that makes it all stay together. Coherence is not the happy inspirational

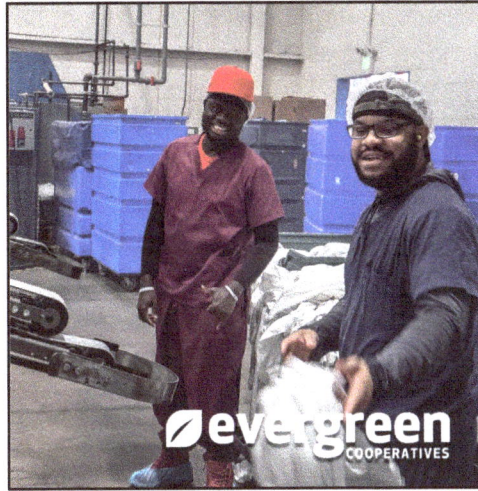
Evergreen Employee Owners
Momar Mbaye & Marvin Minter

part of the story; it explains the toughest, hardest and most foundational part of why it works at all.

This clarity that trustworthiness is related to quality and effectiveness shows up down the road in Dayton which gave birth to flight and, in a more mundane way, many of the key auto parts of the modern era. The starter motor was invented here, so we do not begin our mornings hand cranking our cars.

We were visiting Kettering Health, which has blended faith and healthcare to a very high sustained level, indeed. Once the industrial geniuses of Dayton had begun to succeed with all their inventions and gadgets, they wanted a similarly excellent hospital. They sought out the Adventists, not exactly for religious reasons, but because the Adventists were utterly trustworthy. They were coherent to a very high degree which showed up in how they planned every detail of their hospital services.

They still do and that trust shows up in the hardest of times, when the tornado flattens neighborhoods and the automatic weapon drops surprised people on a festive street. And it is glue when all else falls apart and the schools need serious answers for the fragmented and blown-apart families.

We thought we were just going to meet with a handful of Stakeholder Health friends. But when the subject is faith and the health of the community of Dayton, it turns out that it attracts a stunning roomful of people who want to be part of that story. A story bigger than any one profession, or professional agency or faith tradition, makes possible collaborations that can flex and span the brokenness that would otherwise break all hopes. No Dayton story would resonate without really smart mechanics involved. But everyone these days has plenty of "best practices" they learned from PowerPoints at some meeting.

Here, people like to tinker, figure things out, and then go see if they might fly. They expect failures, but when it is their city and people, they are not going to quit until they figure it out. These days "it" is more likely to involve social, not mechanical arts.

How do we get primary care into the lives of transient young families? The medicine is not that hard, but the really hard part is keeping contact with the kids all the way through school age as they often move multiple times. That looks like a computer data problem, but it really is a human problem of multiple jurisdictions and professions, including the two least transparent of all—healthcare and education.

In Dayton, they have just enough trust among just enough key parts of the structures to have a system that makes it possible to provide continuity of preventive and primary care services from the first contact with the kids in school all the way to graduation.

We learned in a way and methodology you would not expect from people who teach in a school of medicine and university. And we looked at community in a way you would not expect from people who work for large clinical systems of care. So you won't be surprised that we also saw Spirit and the fruits of the Spirit differently than you might expect from Baptists and Methodists. At different stops along road people were more or less comfortable with speaking out of and about their faith.

In Huntington, the Mayor shared his story of making a YouTube plea for prayers in regard to the opioid epidemic. He went so far as to attribute the current reputation of Huntington as a "community of solutions" to prayer. I'm reminded of a cross-knit saying on my office wall: "pray to God, and row toward shore." There have been many, many hands willing to grab an oar and pull hard toward shore. But there have also been many, many prayers.

In Cleveland nobody wanted to talk about Spirit, even the chaplains. But as Fred Smith once noted of Henry Ford Health System, which also rested on an industrial foundation, everyone we met understood they were doing their work with a deep sense it was about way more than their professional interests. And they were deeply confident they had more than their professional cleverness and institutional resources to draw on. That looked like faith then in Detroit, and looks like faith now in Cleveland.

Indianapolis is by far the cleanest big city in the United States. But from the top floors of the shiny buildings downtown you can see neighborhoods that break the heart of anyone who has one. This is where we found Huntington-like quality and tenacity with the same powerful ground game of EMS and former police.

They have, of course, seen everything that others manage to not see, the stuff that would harden anyone's heart. But they do still make eye contact and still their heart is beating. They are glad to work for the church-based community center. They remind me of the story Jesus told of the massive party where nobody important wanted to come. Go to the streets and invite the least to enjoy. The party goes on in East Indianapolis because the invitations are not sent by email, but eye-to-eye.

The heroic nature of the raw responsiveness of the work can mask the thoughtfulness, the systematic planful detail, that enables in-the-moment action. They care enough to think ahead and keep track. They showed up to wish happy birthday to a 94 year-old nearly everyone else forgot. They didn't forget; they wrote it down on their tickler file. Adam's wife made a sign above his door: "When done right, police work looks more like ministry."

What we saw in every stop was a very high order of leadership that was more than problem-solving. We had seen this before in South Africa and were part of a group that created a book that expresses it: "Generative Leadership: Leadership for Turbulent Times." Craig Stewart is a pastor in Cape Town who fits neatly into any one of these tough towns. Trained as a river biologist, he gifted us with a story that I thought of as we drove the rivers of the Inland Sea. A river flows off the cliffs of Table Mountain as it winds seven miles to the ocean. It had been tamed with concrete over the years until it was a 7-mile culvert. How do you bring concrete back to life?

The answer is that you don't have to remove all the damage and restore it. You do have to bore some holes in the bottom so that the life waiting for a chance can explode from the soil. Life rarely misses such a chance and needs little instruction.

So, too, in the bruised towns covered in the concrete glories of an earlier generation. Nobody we spoke to was trying to clear all the left-behind debris, as if it were possible to start entirely fresh. The generative teams of Cleveland, Dayton, Huntington, and East Indianapolis were trying the other approach.

Break a few holes in the hopelessness to give life a chance, and then encourage it. Knock on the door of every overdose survivor and ask if, now

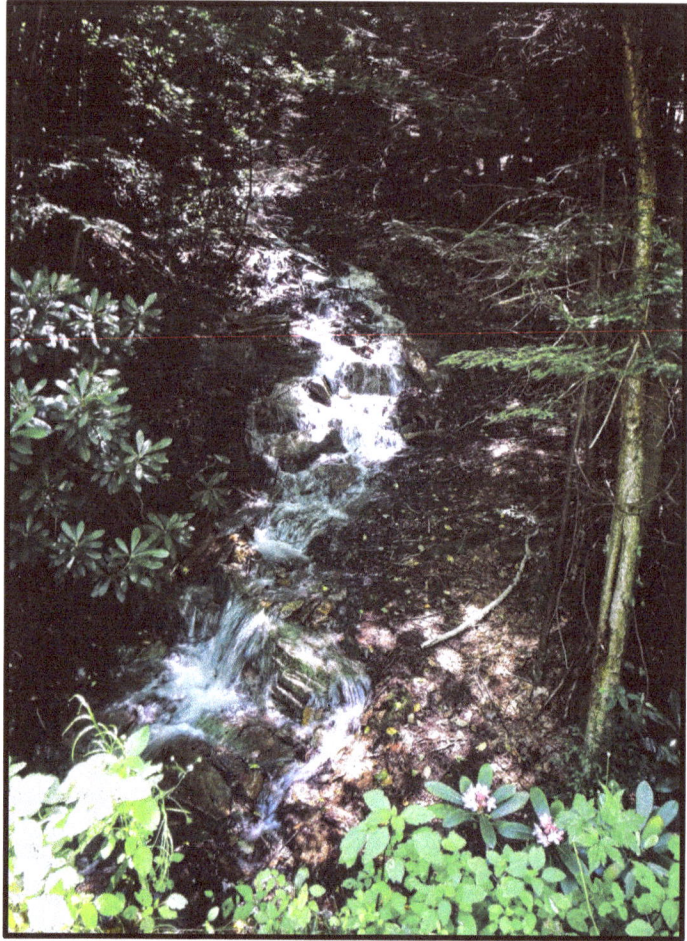

that they are not dead, they want to actually live. That's a pretty radical question, actually, that applies to entire neighborhoods that others not living there might consider beyond hope.

We drove again in a season of intense partisan venom as the impeachment process was underway. We thought that was as bad as it could get, but, of course, we were wrong. No small part of the venom comes wrapped in a weaponized language of faith encouraging and blessing the opposite of the most attractive works of mercy of the saints of Huntington, Cleveland, Dayton, Indianapolis, Bloomington, and points between.

Now that we can see that we're not dead, are we ready to be alive? The evidence to the answer "yes" is very practical and somewhat mundane.

Take one step toward what looks like life. A prayer might be offered, but treatment, too. And a peanut butter sandwich. Then another step. Get someone to walk with you. And then another. Talk to the others moving toward life to see what might be possible in the webs of trust; the practical things like converting a left-behind apartment complex into a home of hope for women who had little reason to expect any. These are very, very practical things by the bushel, and then more, they are like roots finding soil.

The testimony of natural systems is that they don't give up trying and are often rewarded with the most surprising flourishing over time. Why would human systems find their way any other way?

www.ingramcontent.com/pod-product-compliance
Lightning Source LLC
Chambersburg PA
CBHW041911220326
R18017400001B/R180174PG41597CBX00005B/3